PATHWAYS TO PATIENTS

STUDENTS SEEKING MEANING

WJ CRUMP

This book is a testament to the resilience of the patients who invited us into their lives and we acknowledge them and the community physicians who acted as guides. Emma Hampton served as summer student editorial assistant and compiled the large number of essays. Emma Doyle expertly crafted the cover art that conveys exactly what we had hoped. The photo credit, as with all my books, goes to Pam Carter.

SYMBOLISM OF THE COVER

When I was asked to paint the cover art for this book, I thought about what "Pathways to [Reaching] Patients" meant to me. Often our patients are readily reaching out to us, with a vibrant story of their illness and their life leading up to their illness, if only we take the time and energy to listen. With that thought in mind, I was reminded of Michelangelo's "The Creation of Adam." In that painting, Michelangelo portrays God with a fully extended finger reaching to Adam, and Adam with a limp, almost aloof finger, signifying that the Divine is readily available to Adam if only he takes the effort to reach out. In the cover art I decided to reference "The Creation of Adam," positioning a student physician in the place of Adam, meaning that a student needs only to be curious and to listen to find the patient with which they are presented. Learning to reach the patient is the "pathway" to becoming a physician, so I placed a pathway extending from the point at which the student's and patient's fingers should find each other. Above the pathway is a raincloud, which signifies transformation in traditional Western painting, as symbolism of a sort of baptism. If we as medical students learn to find our patients, we are slowly transformed, sometimes in ways that we did not expect, to the empathetic, healing physician that we entered medical school to become in the first place.

Emma Doyle, Trover Rural Campus M-4 Medical Student

PREFACE

There are a great number of books written by practicing physicians recounting the fascinating stories of their patients, and I think I have read most. I've also written several of my own. The inspiration for this collection of patient stories came from my summer sessions with college pre-med students and medical students very early in their training that are called "Friday morning reflections." With no agenda beyond encouraging them to observe their preceptors closely as they interacted with patients, I was struck with how quickly they discovered the power of empathy. They were almost universally impressed with how much each doc knew of their patients' stories, and couldn't imagine how they might do this someday. They also quickly picked up the difference when a doc, usually an "ologist," didn't invest energy in knowing the patient, and the visit was more like an oil change in a quick lube.

Someone early in my career got me keeping a journal and writing patient stories, and after more than 40 years of practice and teaching, it was time to pass it on. In my Associate Dean role at a rural regional medical school campus, I had frequent contact with our third- and fourth-year clinical students. We also had summer programs for carefully selected college students called College Rural Scholars (CRS), a "Prematric" program for students just before they began medical school, and a Preclinical program for students between their first and second year of medical school. As I developed a professional identity curriculum in an attempt to slow the loss in empathy I saw as my graduates began their family medicine residency at our campus, the power of narrative medicine cried out from every reference I found.

On the M-3 Psychiatry clerkship, an essay describing a particularly touching patient interaction was required. I found myself engrossed in these tales, but wishing that there was more depth of understanding of the patient's life prior to the crisis of hospital admission. I found a publication that reported that M-1 medical students tended to report the patient's story, while M-3s were more focused on quickly categorizing the patient's illness into a diagnosis in the current version of whatever coding system was in vogue. In short, curiosity had become replaced by diagnostic efficiency. Knowing that development of this categorization skill was required to be successful during the time crunch of residency training, I set out to provide time and reward for my students at all levels to breathe in the full patient story before it was too late.

The essays in this book are the products of a gentle outline provided to the students to produce a rich patient story given 45 minutes for an interview in a rural clinical environment. As a less structured view, they were also asked to produce a 55-word story about one patient they saw during each precepting session. There are also essays from M-3 students on their Psychiatry clerkship and a few M-4 recollections. Each chapter was carefully curated, but this categorization is more for the casual reader than anything more substantive. Each chapter begins with an essay that provides a broad gestalt of the topic, often by a physician faculty or community practitioner.

The essays are only lightly copy edited, allowing colloquialisms to survive. Almost all the students are themselves from rural Kentucky, and shared idioms were only slightly sifted to more standard usage. Student- assigned pseudonyms or the patient's initials were kept intact, and any potentially identifying information was changed or removed. Almost all essays included the names of the patient's family members and friends, and, remarkably, the names of their pets. These were also anonymized.

These patient stories tell much more about the students' views than just the intricacies of their patients' lives. Even with what some might consider mundane details of everyday Kentucky life, the students discovered the magic of true understanding that is the nidus for empathy. I hope you enjoy them as much as I did.

Bill Crump, M.D.

TABLE OF CONTENTS

Chapter 4: Covid

FOREWORD

IN THE VAST TAPESTRY OF human experiences, there exist stories that are both profound and humble, tales that unfold within the rural corners of our world. Within <u>Pathways to Patients</u>, these narratives are the voices of medical students and rural medical faculty who have traversed the path less taken, discovering a remarkable truth: the challenges they face in underserved areas become the catalyst for personal growth, forging them into new doctors equipped with unparalleled empathy and unwavering determination.

In these pages, students and new doctors embark on a transformative journey where they are welcomed into the lives and hearts of their patients, becoming intertwined in the fabric of their communities. While the details of these stories are changed or omitted to protect patient identities, the core human experience shines through. These accounts show the difficulties and triumphs that shape young doctors, molding them into professionals ready to confront the realities and intricacies of providing healthcare in underserved areas. The profound weight of such encounters elicits deep introspection.

As graduates of the Trover Rural Scholars Program of the University of Louisville, we were fortunate to learn from experienced faculty who taught us how to overcome challenges and provide quality medical care to underserved populations. The program celebrated its 25th anniversary in 2023. Over the years, our fellow graduates have taken the knowledge and skills we gained to rural communities throughout Kentucky and the United States. Many chapters in <u>Pathways to Patients</u> begin with the stories of physicians who have returned to this community in Madisonville, Kentucky, to practice and help teach a new generation of physicians.

This book contains stories of students and young doctors that encapsulate the joy of saving lives, the solace in bringing relief to suffering, and the privilege of supporting populations that are often overlooked. You will also find stories of personal growth that come with the most difficult of experiences, such as in Chapter 3 "Lessons in Resilience." These stories remind us that the rewards of practicing medicine in underserved rural areas extend far beyond professional satisfaction. They breathe life into our collective purpose, reminding us of what we value most.

May these stories inspire and ignite a flame within all who read them, kindling a passion for creating a world where access to quality healthcare knows no boundaries.

Dr. Whitney Gilley and Dr. Reagan Gilley

Regional Affiliate Clinical Faculty, ULSOM Department of Psychiatry and Behavioral Sciences

2013 graduates of ULSOM Trover Rural Track

CHAPTER 1

Initial Impressions Don't Tell the Full Story

PROLOGUE:
WITHOUT DOUBT
WHITNEY GILLEY MD

THE TRAUMA PAGER WENT OFF as I sat alone in the small resident conference room. I was on a pediatric intensive care unit ("ICU") rotation at a rural level one trauma center in the shadow of the Blue Ridge Mountains. This particular pager summoned emergency room physicians and nurses, trauma surgeons, intensivists, and anyone assigned to care for patients whose life would depend on rapid and skilled interventional treatment. As a first-year resident, the sound of the trauma pager set my heart pounding.

I dialed in for the report. A car driven by a female driver, intoxicated on methamphetamine, had crossed over the center of the highway at high speed and collided head-on with an oncoming vehicle. A man was deceased at the scene. Incoming to the trauma bay was the adult female in serious condition and a seven-year-old girl in critical condition. The child was unresponsive and required fluids and pressors to maintain her blood pressure, an ominous sign. The small outlying hospital where both were initially taken had obtained a CT before transferring the child by helicopter to our center.

My role would begin after initial stabilization by the trauma and surgical teams stationed in the ER, and the child brought upstairs to the ICU. I pulled up the patient's chart on the computer to begin to review whatever information had been quickly put together. The head CT was in the system already. I clicked through the first few sections before a wave of nausea struck. Where the spinal cord should connect in one smooth continuation as it enters through the base of the skull, a shadowy interruption lay across the spinal cord where the C1 vertebra meets the base of the skull. It was a full spinal cord transection and incompatible with life.

The neurosurgeon had seen these images too, and determined there was no indication to operate. So not long after the little girl arrived in the emergency department, she was transferred to the pediatric ICU. My purpose was no longer to administer life-saving care, but to keep this child's body alive long enough for her family to say goodbye.

The covering attending was a fearless pediatric ICU fellow nearing the end of her training. She ordered continuous epinephrine by IV to keep the vascular system and heart going in absence of input from the nervous system. I watched the blood pressure and heart rate on the monitor as this slowly became less and less effective.

Over the next few hours, the team began to discuss the logistics of having the now stable mother brought in from her hospital room downstairs. It was important to deliver such painful news in person and give her a few minutes with her daughter. Time was short but so was the staffing needed to move her. To avoid interrupting care of other patients, nursing requested that this be done immediately after the 7am shift change when there would be more nurses available. The ICU physician trade off would occur shortly after this same time, but because the fellow had flown in from the Midwest to provide coverage, she had to make her flight out a little earlier. It would be up to me to deliver the news of the daughters' death to the mother.

Searching for the words to say, I went to stand beside the little girl's bed. From the changes in vascular tone, the face of this child looked so much older than seven. I saw her as a young woman, almost as if she had aged gracefully into her late teens overnight. But she would never become that young woman. Anger flickered up and my cheeks burned. Despite having seen how powerfully the addiction to methamphetamine gripped and destroyed entire communities in Appalachia, despite everything I had learned about addiction as a disease that alters the brain even on a structural level, I could not understand how a mother could do this to her child.

"I'm sorry." I whispered to the little form on the bed.

It is not uncommon for children, and adults, to still love people who hurt them. I wondered if she had loved her mother. I tried to quash the rage threatening to spill over, feeding the thought that yes, her mother needed to see in-person the consequences of what she had done. I had never felt like this before, but it did not change what I needed to do. As a doctor, it wasn't my place to judge, but to try to create something healing out of this--if I could.

In the small pediatric conference room, I sipped a soda and tried to collect myself in the few minutes I had to do so. One of the senior residents knew about the case and must have intuited the weight of this on an inexperienced intern. She looked straight into my eyes.

"I'll talk to the mom." She said.

It wasn't a question, and I did not push back.

We went together to the ICU. A bed with a monitor and IV pole looming over it was parked in front of my patient's room. The glass doors to the ICU rooms retract completely, allowing for equipment to move in and out, or, in this case, to accommodate a hospital bed pulled up alongside. The mother's face was bruised and unreadable. She seemed frozen in place on the bed beneath the bundles of tubes and wires.

The senior resident introduced herself, in a calm, gentle tone that struck awe in me. She explained that the little girl had a severe spinal cord injury high up in her neck, and placed a palm on the woman's gauze wrapped hand in warning of what was coming.

"There is nothing else we can do."

The heart-piercing cry of a mother that has just lost her child is something that cannot be described.

When we arrived back at the conference room, a newspaper lay open on the table to an article about the car crash. The driver who caused the collision while on meth died at the scene. The mother was driving the car with her seven-year-old daughter and had been hit head-on by the other vehicle.

"I was so angry at that mom," the senior resident whispered.

Across the top of the page was a photo of crumpled metal, the objects barely reminiscent of cars. My anger was already spent, and I had none left for the man in the grainy photo in the paper's margin. I wondered at that absence and what else I didn't know about the people I only came to meet beneath the hospital's harsh fluorescent light.

The impact this little girl and her mother had on my practice of medicine continues through to this day. Information is powerful, and in clinical situations we often need it fast. But if the information we receive is incomplete or misunderstood, it can distort the entire picture and lead to wrong conclusions. Embracing curiosity and the truth of uncertainty gives us space for compassion and empathy. I have found this also makes for more astute clinical care. This family taught me that distancing myself from the seductive illusion of certainty is one of the most important skills a physician, and a person, can learn.

DEALING WITH THE BITTERSWEET PATIENTS
ALYSSA HOUNSHELL (MS 3 JULY 2021)

When I first met Joe, he was lying down, his blankets pulled up tightly to cover his face. Taking in this scene, I stepped across the threshold from the bright hallway into his dark room. I reflected back on the notes from his admission I had just been reading. He had been moved involuntarily from the ED to the Behavioral Health Unit after he told the emergency department staff he was going to "blow his head off." I greeted him and asked politely if I could ask him a few questions. He huffed in agreement. As I began asking what had brought him to the BHU, he informed me that all of the information I needed should be in his chart already. Had I even looked at it before I had barged in and interrupted his sleep? Was I stupid or just plain rude? My cheeks reddening under my mask, I assured him that I understood how he felt. "I doubt it," he scoffed, "no one understands the pain I'm going through right now." As the conversation went on, he continually expressed that no one cared for him or listened to him. He lamented that, had he known he would have been placed on an involuntary psychiatric hold, he would have just bought some pain pills from John Doe down the street and never would have come to the hospital in the first place. He repeatedly complained of being "locked up," and rolled his eyes at every empathetic statement I made. With each minute of the agonizing conversation I felt myself shrinking. Maybe if I was lucky, I would disappear altogether. Getting nowhere, I thanked him for his time and left before I agitated him any further. The laid-back introduction I had planned had been turned into what felt like an attack.

Later I would go to let him know that the doctor was ready to see him in the conference room. "You mean I have to walk to him?" he grumbled. I nodded. "Do you need some help sir?" I asked as he slowly stood on unsteady feet. "No I don't need help. Nobody has helped me the whole time I've been here," he spat. I gritted my teeth as he continued to complain as we walked down the hall. My body felt hot and cold all at once. Anger bubbled and then sank like a rock in the pit of my stomach. I felt a pang of guilt, and then shame for how I felt. In the first two years off medical school we had been taught to believe that we would spread joy and love and fix everyone. It would all be sunshine and rainbows. As I entered the conference room filled with dread, Joe sat in his chair as the psychiatrist greeted him. He hunched over, curling his body in on himself, somehow making himself even less approachable. He didn't say a word for a long time. I watched as he clenched his jaw in protest to the onslaught of questions from the doctor. Seconds seemed like hours as we all sat silently awaiting his reply. When he finally spoke, it was clear he was annoyed about having his brain prodded when he felt our goals were much different than his own. "How was your childhood then? Are you perfect?" He hurled his words at the doctor like weapons. I wondered if this is how he talked to everyone. After what seemed like an eternity, the doctor told him he was free to leave, and he slowly rose and staggered back down the hall, muttering profanities with each shaky step. The room collectively let out a sigh of relief, and we were excused for the weekend.

When I arrived on Monday morning, I opened Joe's chart, expecting to see reports that he was guarded and uncooperative throughout the weekend. To my surprise, every note indicated that he had been pleasant. Over the weekend, his KASPER report had come back and it turned out his story about simply not being able to contact his pain management clinic was true. I felt guilt wash over me. I had absolutely pegged this man as a drug seeker, and it turned out he had been truthful throughout his entire stay. He had run out of his pain medication and truly couldn't get an appointment to get them refilled. He had laid at home in pain for a week before he finally arrived in the ER. Hurting so badly that he wished he would just die, he threatened to shoot himself and finally ended up here on the behavioral health unit. I closed the EMR, logged out of the computer and headed to his room. Before I got a chance, I caught a glimpse of him sitting at the end of the hallway, staring out the common room's only window. Early morning sunlight washed over him. In his white shirt and light khaki shorts, it almost looked as if he was glowing. He looked so serene that it seemed impossible that this was the same man who had been so rude to me on Friday. As I approached him, he turned his head to look at me and for the first time, I noticed that his eyes were a rich chocolate brown. "Good morning!" I said, "How are you feeling today?" "Much better," he said with a smile. The wrinkles extending from the corners of his eyes were clues that he had smiled often. His face was kind, cheerful even. I finished my conversation with him and walked over to meet my attending in the conference room. Our first task of the morning was to call and set up a follow-up appointment for Joe at his pain clinic. We called several times and received no answer. We texted the number provided, still with no luck. Finally, my attending decided he would just walk over to the clinic building across the parking lot so they couldn't ignore him any longer. Eventually they did return our call and we got the appointment set up. I went back to find Joe to give him the update, and I told him all about the ordeal. "It looks like you all got a taste of what I was dealing with," he laughed. We talked for a few more minutes, and I wished him well as I said goodbye to him for the last time before he was discharged.

Joe was the first patient to push me to the point of anger. He was the first patient I saw who made me feel like a nuisance, the first to yell at me, and the first to refuse my help. As much as I struggled having Joe as my patient, he taught me perhaps the most important lesson a medical student can learn. We see patients at their worst. We see the messy, ugly, raw reality of pain and suffering. Often, we see patients who have fallen through the cracks. His behavior was not an indication that he was a bad person. Instead, it was a cry for help from a man in misery. Joe may have been the first patient to make me angry, but he was also the first patient to make me feel truly fulfilled. I hope I never forget him.

DID HIGH SCHOOL FOOTBALL CAUSE PSYCHOSIS? BLAKE EDMONSON (PRE-MATRIC JUNE 2020)

Conversing with someone who is actively in psychosis is something that has fascinated me for years. Many of my preconceptions about these patients have stemmed from television shows or books, but I never was able to truly know what it would be like. My first reaction upon entering the psych unit of the hospital was sort of unsettling. It was hard to grasp the idea that these patients were like me in many ways but have deeper, physical imbalances that were out of their control. I was able to sit down and converse with a schizophrenic patient, Mr. S. I was very nervous about this interaction as my preconceptions about schizophrenic patients being "crazy" started to take over. However, I quickly learned that he was a very normal person who has just dealing with his own problems.

Mr. S was a very young patient, age 25, and was very open to talking with me about the "voices" that continue to bring toil into his life. He was a relatively skinny man who had personally shaved his head and part of his eyebrows. His physical appearance was very similar to the main character of the movie *Split*. However, he did not possess multiple personalities like that figure. We began by discussing his past and family. He informed me that he was from an area about an hour and half away from the hospital and has been back and forth since graduating high school. He has two sisters and one brother who are all younger than him. He relayed to me that football was what he missed the most about high school. He talked about how it gave him a purpose. He loved the commitment to the sport, the conditioning, the weightlifting, and the physical contact. He even stated that he was a defensive tackle despite his smaller frame. He claimed that he played every snap of every game on offense and defense. He believes he received numerous concussions from this, and these were the start of his issues.

So far, my conversation with Mr. S was casual and mild. However, it became much more vocal when discussing the reason why he was in the hospital. I was very nervous about asking about his psychological issues as I was afraid to trigger something. I spoke very softly and asked broadly about his conditions. He was quick to state that the "Chinese" were out to get him. He stated that there is a voice of a Chinese girl that is constantly yelling negative things in his right ear. He says that she is very loud and evil. I was completely at a loss on how to respond to this. I was unable to empathize or even relate his story to another case. I remained quiet and let him continue to talk. He then stated that there is another voice of a young "Mexican" boy who also yells negative things at him. These voices drive him to think about crazy things and make him paranoid all the time. He claims that the Chinese are out to invade the United States and even target him specifically for an unknown reason. Hearing all of this made me feel like I was on a television show like Criminal Minds. His condition and story were unlike anything I had personally experienced and felt like a made-up scenario. I was very intrigued by this conversation, and my preconceptions about these types of patients were lifted. Our conversation ended soon after his explanations of his "voices". I thanked him for his time, and we parted ways. I believe this conversation was very educational and eye-opening for me.

JUST ANOTHER DEPRESSED PATIENT
TRAVIS WHEELER (MS 4 OCTOBER 2014)

I had interacted with schizophrenic patients in the past, but the patients I had seen in the past were not actively psychotic. From the outside Anne looked like any other working class middle-aged woman. Throughout the interview I was having a rather heated internal emotional battle between sympathy and amazement. Perhaps such a battle reflects my naivety as a young medical student, but I had never seen a patient with a presentation such as Anne's.

My sense of sympathy came from the obvious fact that Anne had no insight into what was wrong. She seemed frustrated that other people wouldn't believe what she was saying. She wasn't upset because she was having uncontrollable and preposterous thoughts that were out of touch with reality; to her she was not sick. She was trapped in her reality where no one understood her, no one believed her, and no one would help her.

In conflict with my sense of sympathy was a sense of amazement. We often see television representations of real life that are not quite accurate. While listening to Anne talk about her plans to visit the president, and the modification of human beings to subsist on their own secretions I found myself in shock of how much her presentation was like that of not only various television depictions but also medical text books. In most cases the Hollywood version is exaggerated and fictionalized and I assumed that it would be true in the case of a patient suffering from Schizophrenia. On the contrary, her thoughts were just as, if not more, extravagant as what we see on TV or in film; she could easily have just stepped off of the set of the latest silver screen drama and into the waiting room.

In looking back on this experience, perhaps the most obvious lesson I will take from it is to be more careful not to "judge a book by its cover." My initial impression on seeing Anne was that she was just another depressed patient. While my assumption was quickly shattered upon the start of the encounter, I could easily apply this lesson to a variety of other situations. As a physician I must not be too quick to come to a conclusion about a patient.

Additionally, I gained a better understanding of chronic mental illness. On various other rotations I have seen countless patients with chronic medical conditions. The diabetic patient is well aware that their body has a problem utilizing the sugar they consume. They understand that in order to maintain their health and prevent the progression of their illness it is necessary to eat a specific diet and to get plenty of exercise, whether they do it or not. In the case of chronic mental illness however, particularly those such as schizophrenia, the patient is unaware that anything is wrong. They don't understand why their doctor is telling them to take medication, or why everyone thinks they are crazy.

It was both enlightening and humbling to speak with Anne and to see a prime example of the limitations of the practice of medicine. Doctors are expected to treat illnesses and to fix people, but the simple fact is that for some people and some illnesses little can be done until they begin to see their condition as needing fixing. I don't know that I had ever truly embraced such an idea until I spoke with Anne.

LOCKING AWAY TRAUMA
KELSEY WILLEN (MS 4 NOVEMBER 2015)

I reflected on a visit with an attractive older woman who had a warm feeling about her as if she could have been one of my grade school teachers. However, as the patient told her story, a truly tragic series of events unfolded, including childhood sexual abuse. She felt abandoned by her mother who didn't believe her reports of the abuse by her step-father, and she married the "love of her life" in her teens to get out of this situation. Then her husband met a tragic death. And most of this story was being told for the first time to anyone.

After the patient explained what was troubling her, the interview room had a palpable feeling of sadness. I worried that discussing such tragic memories would make her depression worsen. However, her face now showed a sign of peace as she told us, "I'm relieved finally to talk to some-one about these terrible things I've kept locked away for so long."

This experience not only changed my understanding of her, but also impacted how I will treat patients in the future. My first impression of her only revealed a superficial coating, an act to hide the dark layers and depth of her life. I was fortunate enough to be able to learn about her past and what makes her the depressed, anxious person she is today. The doctor-patient relationship is such an important factor and without trust and understanding a doctor is just treating an illness, not a person. Once a doctor has that connection he or she can begin to ask the difficult questions that might not always be comfortable, but are necessary. I am saddened that she waited over 40 years to reveal these deplorable stories, but am glad that she was willing to open up to me. I will remember this patient interaction when I am a practicing physician and hope that my patients will feel comfortable enough and trusting of me to tell me sensi-tive information. I will also remember never to judge or assume someone is fine just by his or her outward appearance, because he or she could be hurting inside and actually really seeking the opportunity to talk to someone.

TREMORS
LINDSAY TUCKER (CRS JULY 2021)

As we walked in, her hand shaking, I could sense the anxiety she was feeling. It wasn't until she pulled down her mask that I see this tremor was more than just nervousness. However, her new medication wasn't the cause, so a CT was ordered and we moved on. I wonder how she is now.

A TROOPER WITH A HEART
CIERRA WOODCOCK (CRS JULY 2020)

Mr. M is an older gentleman from really small town, Kentucky. He came in for a regular checkup to discuss his uncontrolled diabetes and love for chocolate. He was otherwise very healthy and had no other issues. Walking in, it was easy to see that he was quiet and had reservations about a 20-year-old student asking him questions about his life. Nonetheless, he provided some insight into what his life looked like over the years.

He served as a state trooper for 27 years, until his retirement in 1984. After his retirement as a trooper, he became a part of the narcotics task force and began handling white-collar crimes. He mentioned that he chose to retire from being a state trooper because the amount of murders he had to deal with did not set well with him. He then discussed how the white-collar crimes he had dealt with for the last 17 years rarely involved murders, but large amounts of cash and drugs. He stated that the amount of money and drugs he had witnessed as an officer working narcotics was not like anything any normal civilian could ever imagine. At this moment in time, it was easy to see that Mr. M was holding back some information, things that he probably did not feel comfortable discussing with someone not familiar with law enforcement. With a sigh he said, "A lot of people just don't understand what it is like to be an officer of the law." He did not believe that a student could ever understand what the life of a law enforcement officer was like. In an attempt to relate to Mr. M, I mentioned that my significant other was a law enforcement of-ficer and there were many days that I witnessed first-hand what being an officer looked like. In that exact moment, Mr. M had a total change in attitude. His eyes lit up, and a large smile came across his face; someone understood. Details began to flood out of him like a river. He mentioned shootings that he had been involved in, protecting minorities and members of the LGBTQ+ community, politics, teaching a gun safety course, and how each of them affected him personally over the years. Ending the discussion, the conversation shifted from light and exciting to serious. He opened up about how he had gotten a divorce only 4 years after becoming an officer, due to his own mistakes. He said that over the years, he has watched many young officers make the same mistakes and lose their partners. He hated seeing officers and their partners go through what he had to. He left me with a simple piece of advice: "in life, you will witness many things that will disturb you, especially as an officer. Do not hold it all in and shut those you love the most out; let them in. Communication is key in every successful relationship, and if you let the ones you love in, they will never fail you and the two of you will live a happy life."

Once Mr. M knew that I understood what that aspect of his life entailed, and that I was on his side, the relief he felt was visible and it was clear that being a police officer was his biggest passion in life. Witnessing his shift in attitude was one of the most amazing things that I have ever experienced. I was even more amazed by the advice he gave me about communication and letting people in. It was easy to see that those words came from a place of love and kindness. What began as an encounter with a tough guy, ended with a kind man that wanted to help someone in a situation similar to his own. As a future physician, this demonstrated that first impressions are not always what they seem and sometimes it just takes someone knowing that you understand and are on their side. At the end of the day, it is the doctor and patient versus the problem, not the doctor versus the patient.

THE ALCOHOLIC BORDERLINE AND ME
ANNILIN SEVERNS (MS 3 OCTOBER 2016)

The morning started with a text from my attending saying, "the famine is over; the feast has begun." I was excited. It had been so slow. It was full moon. In a matter of hours, the small Madisonville inpatient unit flooded with eight new patients. The two weeks prior capped census at approximately five patients total. Now, we were up to twelve under the solo care of the psychiatrist and his trusty (and humble) side kick, me. I eagerly dressed and rushed out the door. My thoughts raced manically through the possibilities of who could be behind those doors. Who was I going to meet today? How would I decide which patient to see first? Maybe I'll even meet a patient I could write my reflection paper on...

Julie is a bipolar alcoholic hospitalized for suicidal ideation. Her past medical history landed her in the hospital for a couple of days, but an alcohol withdrawal seizure led her to the 6th floor for psychiatric help. Her medical history includes alcoholic hepatitis and cirrhosis and she is currently taking opiate pain medication for back pain from a past car wreck. That vignette alone draws a very negative picture. Alcoholic with pain pills and liver cirrhosis—if this were a question stem, it would get a resounding eye roll by most medical students. But psychiatry pushes deeper than what's written on someone's chart, lab tests, and medications. It goes more in depth than a 10 minute conversation with your primary care doctor. Psychiatry takes this black and white drawing of diagnostic criteria and transforms it into a colorful work of art.

Julie began drinking at 5 years old. Unsurprisingly in the world of psychiatry, this began secondary to childhood abuse. Her mom would give her alcohol to loosen her up for her drinking buddies. The abuse started after her father committed suicide; she found him hanging over her bed at four years old. For the next 10 years, she lived in a sexually, physically, verbally, and emotionally abusive household where alcohol was her crutch. Now, in the psychiatry unit, multiple people were asking about her past—a past that she repressed for years—and she was forced to reckon with these emotions without the numbing effect of alcohol. If she didn't wake up tomorrow, she would be fine with that.

Julie and I would catch up every day throughout her stay. She would complain about her medications and how she felt. I would talk to her and calm her down. She was agitated, emotional, and frustrated that she was feeling for the first time in 30 years. Frustrated and overwhelmed, she once said, "I've heard him say something about Latuda...latude me!" She always said funny, lighthearted things like that (another example was calling Geodon shots the "booty juice" shot), pausing the interview for us to laugh. There were times randomly in the middle of the day she'd see me and ask to talk. I'd sit there and just listen. She knew I had no control of her medications, but she still wanted to talk to me.

The entire time it seemed like she had been straight with me. We made many medication adjustments, hesitant sometimes with her history of alcoholism and concurrent use of opiate pain medications. She insisted repeatedly, "I don't have a pill problem, I have a drinking problem! I am a drunk!" At the end of her stay, with her medications adjusted, she was ready for discharge. I made sure to see her before I left that day and she hugged me goodbye.

The day after she was discharged, I learned she was back in the hospital. The report said she had suffered a seizure. Alcohol and urine toxicology screen were clean. No other notes had been dictated at the time I looked through her chart. The least I could do was go touch bases with her. Her eyes lit up when she saw me and she quickly pulled me in the room and explained to her fiancé I was "one of the good ones." I listened closely to her recap of the past 12 hours or so and realized the central subject—Ativan. Although the psychiatrist had initially refused to prescribe Ativan, her anxiety and agitation (and potentially her manipulative story telling nature) eventually warranted some Ativan prescribed. The discharging physician did not include that in her discharge medications. How was she not supposed to have an alcohol withdrawal seizure (10 days sober) without her prescription of Ativan, she demandingly questioned me.

She painted a nice story for me. There had been three different physicians managing the psychiatry unit in four days. I'm sure she may have convinced someone to give her more Ativan than the original doctor advised. She was discharged by a new physician with who she was unfamiliar. She explained to me that she felt discarded and neglected. However, the root of these feelings were tied up the absence of a prescription. I listened to her list her complaints about everything from the medicines to the doctors and how she was never coming back to this hospital again. I apologized as I had to leave to go to a class and told her I was sorry things were not working out like she wanted, but that I hoped she would get better.

About an hour later, I talked to the psychiatry nurse practitioner to ask about what had happened with discharging Julie. The nurse practitioner had run a KASPER and found numerous instances of doctor and pharmacy shopping. Her story started falling apart. She hadn't been in Madisonville by chance. She did in fact have a problem with pills. She was not interested in getting better.

My whole body sighed. I had spent an entire weekend worrying about how she was doing. She was the patient I eagerly woke up to go see and catch up on the events of the night. I advocated for her needs when I presented to the psychiatrist. She just seemed misunderstood. She seemed like someone who needed help. But in reality, she just needed someone to help her get some benzodiazepines until the next time.

I got manipulated by a borderline patient and that made me so incredibly angry with myself and her. I was mad that I didn't use more precaution. I was upset that I believed her. I was livid that I spent so much time thinking about her. I was disappointed that I went to check on her when I saw she had been readmitted. But that's psychiatry.

Psychiatry isn't a field where I got to pick the colors I was going to use to color in Julie's diagnostic drawing. As much as I tried to manipulate Julie's story and turn it into a childhood trauma turned alcoholic who confided in me her desire to get better, the colors weren't there. That makes psychiatry beautiful. It involves creativity, time, thoughtfulness, and perseverance. Psychiatry involves understanding and acceptance that there will not be a completed masterpiece at the end of each patient encounter. In Julie's story, I didn't even come close to coloring anything in, but I tried.

A patient eliciting this series of emotions can only be reflected upon as positive. Getting mad at a patient means I care. My future career as a physician will not have a 100% success rate in treating and curing patients from disease. Patients will lapse and fall off the wagon. But, the second I don't get upset or angry with them or myself is the second I need to reevaluate who I am becoming. Borderline or not, each patient deserves an ear to be heard and a physician who believes in them. That's the lesson I choose to take from Julie. That's how I choose to move forward, and I thank her for that.

A FLOWER-GARDENING NANA WITH SPUNK
EMMA DOYLE (PRE-MATRIC JUNE 2020)

On my second morning of preceptorship for pre-matriculation, I am sent to the residency clinic at the local hospital. I am shown to a long corridor-like room with desks and computers lining the walls. Every station represents a resident, and without counting, there seem to be about twenty residents working at the clinic. I am introduced to Dr. G who is seated directly right of the door that leads to the exam rooms. After explaining my assignment to Dr. G, she suggests that I interview her first patient of the day, Mrs. J, as she points to Mrs. J's chart on her monitor. Mrs. J has been experiencing a chronic cough from a case of bronchitis for the last few months and has a history of asthma, pleurisy, and leukemia.

When Mrs. J arrives, Dr. G and I both adjust our face shields over our surgical mask-covered faces and make our way down the hall to the appropriate exam room. Mrs. J is sitting in a chair with her purse seated next to her in the next chair. Dr. G introduces me as a new medical student, a thought that gives me momentary emotional whiplash, and asks if it would be alright if I talked with her a while. Mrs. J agrees, and I take a seat in a stool opposite her chair and ask me to tell me anything she would like the doctor to know about her, medically-related or not.

Mrs. J immediately opens the floodgates to talk about her cough; she is understandably exasperated. As I knew already, Mrs. J explains to me that she has been coughing since early March and that whatever she does, she cannot find relief. She was also experiencing a low-grade fever at that time, which made her seek professional care for the first time in more than a year. Mrs. J. was tested twice for influenza, but both tests came back negative. The doctor suspected that Mrs. J. had COVID-19, but no test for the virus was available to the hospital at that time. Mrs. J. was given several antibiotics for bronchitis and was sent home under quarantine for good measure.

Mrs. J's cough did not improve, and in early May she decided to seek care again. She was tested for COVID-19 this time, but the test came back negative. The doctor decided to prescribe Mrs. J. a Medrol steroid pack to help subside her cough. Mrs. J. improved greatly over the next few hours, and she began working in her flower garden for the first time in months while only experiencing a few light chest aches. By morning, however, Mrs. J. began coughing again, coupled with pain in her lungs. Mrs. J went back to the doctor that day. This time an X-ray was ordered to check for pneumonia, but the X-ray did not show any signs of fluid in her lungs. Mrs. J. was prescribed a stronger antibiotic, which at least made the lung pain more light.

When all is said and done, Mrs. J tells me she is simply tired of her cough. While completing the smallest of tasks, or even talking or standing, Mrs. J finds breathing increasingly difficult. Sitting still is the only time when Mrs. J feels any relief. As a result, Mrs. J. has had to give up many of her favorite pastimes. Before the cough, Mrs. J enjoyed tending to her garden, fish pond and shade trees. When I ask her to tell me more about her garden, Mrs. J recalls a tornado in 2005 that blew over two of her shade trees, one of which fell onto her house. She tells me that now she often prays for the health of her remaining trees. Once, Mrs. J tried to grow veggies in her garden, but Japanese beetles wreaked havoc over them as if the leaves had been "beaten up." Now, Mrs. J has given up raising vegetables and sticks to growing lilies instead. Since the cough, though, Mrs. J has been unable to tend to her garden without shortness of breath and fatigue. All of the fish in the pond have died and the flower beds have grown up with weeds. Her husband encourages Mrs. J to sit out on the porch to at least get out of the house, but Mrs. J cannot enjoy the fresh air without fretting over the disarray of her garden. To avoid worrying, Mrs. J opts to stay indoors.

Outside of tending her garden, Mrs. J tells me she misses singing in her band. When she was younger, Mrs. J became a fan of AC/DC and became a heavy-metal singer at the age of eighteen. Mrs. J boasts that at one point she could scream a high F sharp. Now, she is a member of a heavy metal band with her husband, who is a fellow musician. Unfortunately, Mrs. J's cough has impeded upon her singing. Mrs. J looks forward to the day when she continue making music with her bandmates.

Although Mrs. J was never confirmed to have COVID-19, she continues to take special precautions to lower the risk of infecting her family with the virus. Before the pandemic, Mrs. J loved to dote on her grandchildren and be their "nana." Now, with both the COVID-19 outbreak going on and with Mrs. J's ceaseless cough, she has not seen her grandchildren in quite some time. Mrs. J bought some ingredients to bake her grandchildren some chocolate chip cookies, but her cough has robbed her of the energy she needs to make them. Mrs. J shakes her head and tells me that the flour and sugar are still sitting on her kitchen counter, collecting dust.

When asked what she would like to have in her future, Mrs. J. sighs and tells me she hopes to become as fit as she was when she was younger. With a tiny chuckle, Mrs. J mentions that she wishes she weighed 140 pounds again. Aside from her goal weight, Mrs. J misses running and biking and wishes she could run or bike anywhere she wants without coughing. Mostly, she misses the freeing feeling of spending time exercising outdoors and generally feeling healthy.

I thank Mrs. J for her time, and Mrs. J wishes me luck in school with a reassuring smile in her eyes. I leave the room and make my way back to the Computer Corridor to organize my notes. I realize that, when I first saw Mrs. J, I never would have imagined that she was a heavy metal screamer. Obviously I have some stereotypes built up in my mind that are not always accurate. As I scribble some lines and arrows in my notes, I quietly remind myself that I will never know what a person is like until I start to talk with them.

THE ROAD OUT OF DEPRESSION
SHANNON FOSTER (MS 3 JULY 2017)

I was sent downstairs to the medicine ward for a new psychiatric consult. I saw Donna, a 56 year old woman, sitting in a hospital gown with her sister nearby and the "sitter" at the door to make sure Donna did not hurt herself. After introductions, it was quite clear that Donna wasn't in the mood to speak with anyone. She only wanted 3 things: a cigarette, someone to say she could go home, and her husband. Her husband had died 11 months ago after many months of struggle with cancer.

Donna had tried to kill herself by cutting her wrists, after two more recent deaths in the family had driven her into a dark depression. She had been taking Zoloft for depression since her husband's death but glared at me and angrily responded that she didn't need therapy when I asked. I decided to cut the interview short, to avoid upsetting her further and unnecessarily.

A little later, I returned with our psychiatrist. He began in on his questions and received similarly short, emotional answers. When asked about therapy, Donna pointed at her sister and said that she was her therapy and glared as hard as she could at the doctor. He explained to Donna that she would need to be admitted upstairs on the psychiatric ward, and Donna lost it. She started screaming, "No, no, no!" and turned to her sister, "Don't let them take me!" Our doctor explained the sister didn't have a say in it, and Donna threw off the blankets, screamed that she wouldn't go, and attempted to leave. Between the sitter blocking the doorway and security being called to help, Donna was coaxed down and given sedatives for the transfer. Between sobs, she glared at me and our doctor as hard as she could.

The next morning, the inpatient psychiatric treatment team met to discuss Donna's case and discussed her emotional state at the time of admission and possible ways forward for her. Donna had been asleep throughout the night and was able to dress herself and eat breakfast before meeting with us. She hadn't slept well at all for the 11 months since her husband's death.

When Donna met with us, we started as usual by introducing ourselves and our role in her treatment team. When I spoke, she made eye contact but began to shake very slightly and looked worried. When our doctor introduced himself, she broke into apologies between sobs and gasps. She remembered the events of the day prior and felt horrible for acting out, explaining that she was just "so angry." She hadn't ever faced or dealt with her husband's death. They had been the best of friends for a 36 year marriage, and she did not realize how far she had traveled into depression until she hit the bottom. Our doctor's response was what she needed to hear, "Well, this is the place to express your emotions. We're all here to help you."

Over just a couple of days of therapy, medication, counseling, and activities on the ward, Donna was unrecognizable. She walked taller, she smiled, she held conversations, and she thanked us for being supportive and helpful. She knew the road out of depression was just starting, and it wasn't going to be short or easy, but she realized how far her life had changed for the worse in 11 months, and she wanted a good life back, even if it had to be without her husband. She told us that she just hadn't realized how deep she had slipped as time went by over those months until she was placed on the ward and out of her usual environment to see more clearly where she was emotionally.

I was shocked at my own transformation in those few days. My attitude and view of Donna had turned around as well. Initially on the medicine ward, I saw a lady that was obviously depressed but out of control, dramatic, and maybe even psychotic, and I remember wondering if she was on drugs. Now all I saw was her pain, her suffering, her immense strength in trying to hold on all by herself without putting any of her needs on her children or grandchildren. I saw so much potential and hope from her and for her. She had changed from "a psych consult on the 4th floor" to Donna, a person with a life and family and problems that she needed some help with.

While I don't think I felt anything negative towards her on first impression, I certainly hadn't taken time to consider all the possible things she was dealing with (or more accurately hadn't dealt with) that had led to her hospitalization to begin with. I now more easily see patients with the idea that there's a story and a lifetime of history behind their reason for being in the hospital. Whether it's a psychiatric patient or not, that's true for everyone. Every part of a person's life influences their health and well-being, whether it is physical, social, environmental, economic, or otherwise. Remembering that will help in understanding the patient's situation more fully, which I hope will guide me in developing a better possible treatment plan with them that addresses as many road blocks to recovery as possible.

THE STUDIOUS OBSERVER
EMMA DOYLE (PRE-MATRIC JUNE 2020)

When I started my first morning of precepting in the psychiatric ward, I noticed Ms. V silently watching me from the end of the common room.

She was sitting alone next to a small side table, back of the chair against the wall. She had long, gorgeously curly black hair that fell just below her chest and was wearing a Nike leopard-print active wear shirt and pants set, dazzling high-saturation blue nail polish, and the same neon yellow socks with treads that I assumed every patient was given. She probably stood out to me because she was about my age, unlike many of the much older patients on the adult ward. She also had a striking resemblance to a painter I knew from the art school whose expertise was in mimicking botanicals in her paintings.

Upon introducing myself to Ms. V and explaining my project to her, Ms. V expressed to me that she was uncomfortable disclosing any information about herself to me, saying that she wanted to protect her privacy and only talk with doctors. I completely understood; I was not sure that I would want to intimately discuss my life with a brand new med student either. I thanked her for her time, and we exited the conference room together. The psychiatric nurse practitioner on the ward noticed us leaving, approached us, and asked Ms. V what was the matter. After a few short moments of gentle persuasion, Ms. V agreed to speak with me as long as we did not discuss her prior health history and if the APRN stayed in the room with us. The new group of three reentered the conference room and I initiated the interview.

Ms. V lives with her family, whom she declined to give me details about when asked. She has no hobbies to speak of. Instead, Ms. V has spent a great deal of her life in school. She says that most schooling, whether it be elementary school, high school, college, or beyond, is all just a continued repetition of learning the same few topics over and over again. Ms. V remembers first studying criminal justice, after which she attended culinary school. Culinary school was difficult for Ms. V because she was and is a vegan, she believes strongly that "animals are not here to be eaten." Ms. V refuses to cook or eat any animals or animal products or even fruit; she sticks to eating vegetables only, and likes to eat them especially when they are steamed. Ms. V also learned in culinary school about various diseases animal products can be infected with, which has led her to research the contents of prescription drugs. She has found that many medicines are made with animal products and now refuses to take those drugs. Ms. V even talks to other patients about their drugs to make sure that they know where their prescriptions come from as well.

When I ask Ms. V about any work she has done, she tells me that she has a long history of working in a local daycare as the assistant principal. She never was given much opportunity to work with children at the daycare; she says her job mostly involved desk-work, including answering the telephone and doing paperwork. Ms. V tells me, however, that she was able to form some close attachments with a few of the children. Ms. V recalls one child fondly that did not want to return home to see his mother, that he tried their hardest to stay in the office with Ms. V. Ms. V says that she grew very close to the children and thought of them as her own.

Toward the end of the interview, Ms. V asked me what I was going to school for and what career I wanted. I told her I was interested in psychiatry. Ms. V told me that psychiatry was certainly an interesting field and that she remembered studying psychology herself in college. Most of her studies were online, which she hated. Ms. V remembers figuring out when and where psychology courses met to sit outside the lecture hall to be able to hear what was being said and take notes. Ms. V notices that I am taking notes on a pad and says that using paper to study will help me greatly. Ms. V knows a lot about psychiatry, and she is kind enough to offer me some advice. She reminds me to study hard and to be careful about the things I say and do.

Ms. V is usually a quiet person, but not because she is aloof. Ms. V tells me she is quiet because she is always observing her surroundings, especially people's facial expressions and body language. She says this has made her an unusually empathetic person even though she might not always show it. I realize that must have been why I noticed Ms. V watching me earlier in the morning.

To conclude the interview, I ask Ms. V what she would like her life to look like when she leaves the hospital. After a moment of silent reflection, she tells me that she would like to go back to work, but this time in an elementary school rather than a daycare. She says that moving up the promotion ladder in her field of work is difficult, but she would like to start work in a brand new place. I wish Ms. V luck in the future, thank her for her time, and we silently leave the room accompanied by the quietly watchful APRN so that Ms. V can get on with her day.

UNEXPECTED
MCKINLEY HEFLIN (MS 3 NOVEMBER 2015)

When C.W. walked into the room, I immediately tried to diagnose him. He was younger, well kept, composed, and seemed to be a regular, every day, normal guy. Based on my previous experiences in the psychiatry office, I put on my thinking cap and immediately nailed the diagnosis of ADHD without needing to hear one word from the patient. I relaxed into my seat, smirking to myself at my detective skills, and thought I knew everything that would be said during the visit.

I was wrong. C.W. was twenty-two years old and had a long history of psychiatric problems dating back to the age of six. He had obedience trouble in school most of his life, had been expelled once for bringing a knife to school, and had been in jail for many minor offenses. However, that was just the tip of the iceberg on what I was unable to conceive with my quick, poor, diagnostic judgment before the interview began. C.W. had also been previously diagnosed with schizophrenia. He had such horrible delusions and hallucinations that he was admitted to Western State Hospital on three different occasions and two other psychiatric programs in other parts of western Kentucky.

I sat in awe as the psychiatrist asked C.W. to fill me in on his diverse history of problems with the law, experiences in different institutions, and a stint when he was homeless. I was baffled at how the person who sat calm, cool, and collected in front of me could have endured so many harsh experiences at such a young age. Then he continued to amaze me as he explained his future plans. He was currently taking classes to get his GED and passionately described how he longed to go to culinary school. He spoke with such gusto about his last cooking experience that it actually left me salivating.

C.W. dumbfounded me that day. I know that physicians strive to help their patients to improve their lives, but his physicians, psychologist, and counselors had worked together in order to literally turn this young man's life around. No amount of studying from textbooks, lectures, or online videos can show you how much of an impact the correct medications, listening, effort, and willingness to help can have on a person. His whole life had been changed.

This encounter left me feeling blessed to be part of a profession that can make such a huge impact on the lives of others. I do not know how many hours of therapy, counseling, and different medication combinations were tried to find the perfect combination, but it left me feeling inspired by the system of medical professionals that worked together to help C.W. not only become a productive member of society, but for him to have the potential to reach his dreams. However, I also felt ashamed of myself. I had been quick to judge a person by their outward appearance. I learned that as a future physician this is something that I will not accept. You can never truly know what each person is going through. Every patient is a unique person and is going through a struggle. I need to be able to treat every patient with equal respect and truly listen to what they have to say, instead of hastily jumping to conclusions of what I believe to be considered textbook.

BEING THE EXAMPLE
SHAINA MAGNESS (PRE-MATRIC JULY 2022)

The patient was voluntarily admitted to inpatient psychiatry (6E) because she felt like her life was falling apart and she couldn't handle it all on her own anymore. A series of life-altering events triggered her already anxious personality into full blown panic attacks that prevented her from living her life. She even had trouble sleeping because her thoughts wouldn't stop. Some days she said she felt like she needed to get in her car and drive far away, abandoning all the responsibilities she has undertaken, but she is a very caring mother and daughter, so she continued to put others' needs first. Throughout the conversation it was very evident that throughout her life, she had always put so much towards taking care of everyone else that somewhere along the way she forgot to take care of herself. She doesn't have any hobbies, and even though she used to love camping and hiking, she hasn't gone in years.

The patient's daughter was diagnosed with schizophrenia at age eighteen and she has continued to live with her mother ever since, the court entrusting her to be her daughter's legal caretaker indefinitely. It has been rough. She was isolated due to her daughter's condition for several years, unable to do anything outside of the house besides work. But she learned the ins and outs of schizophrenia treatment and has ensured her daughter received the best treatment available. However, now, at thirty-six, her daughter is more stable and ready to live her own life. Her daughter recently moved four hours away to live with her boyfriend and attend vocational school, leaving the patient with an empty nest for the first time. She wants to let her daughter experience her own life, but she is so scared of her daughter being treated harshly and relapsing into an unhealthy mental state. In addition to this, the patient also had to face living her own life now, one that doesn't revolve around her daughter and her needs, which is stressful in its own right.

Around the same time, a car accident injured her, her mother, and her sister. She now suffers from chronic pain in her right shoulder and hip. While receiving treatment for the accident, she was diagnosed with lung cancer. Even though her cancer was removed with a lobectomy, she was confronted with her own mortality and forced to consider how she wanted to live the rest of her life and how she would leave others if she were gone. In addition to this, she became the primary caregiver for her mother whose mental and physical condition declined following her accident-related injuries. She couldn't rely on her out-of-state brothers to assist with the care of her mother, nor her sister. It's hard to reverse roles and undertake the care of one's parent, but on top of everything else, it began to wear on her until she felt like she couldn't handle any of it anymore.

So, she willingly went to the hospital to try to get help and set an example for her daughter. She wanted to feel better and prove that it is ok to seek mental help when you really need it. I think she is an intelligent, caring woman who is trying her best and I hope she learns from her stay in 6E that she deserves to take care of herself just as much as she takes care of others. Hopefully she can learn what it means to live the life she wants and go camping once more.

When asked if there was anything she wanted people to consider when thinking of herself or others who struggle with their mental health, she explained how mental disorders and poor mental health can have an outstanding effect on not only the patient, but everyone around them. She implores others to treat people with kindness because you never know what struggles they may be facing.

ABUSE ON AISLE 3
NIKKI HARNAGE (CRS JULY 2023)

I clutched the patient list in my hands as I rounded the common area where the patients gathered for the last bits of breakfast. Calling out the name I was assigned to interview, the only response I received was an absent point. As I followed along the bony finger to across the room, my eyes landed on a young woman talking over the counter of the nurse's station. I was struck by her kept hair and clothes. She wore black jeans and a long sleeve with a Japanese cartoon cat—a marked difference from the blue paper scrubs most of the patients opted for. I was struck by just how *average* she was.

As I called her name, she turned and her eyes and smile lit up. The absurd thought that she belonged in Walmart and not here popped into my mind. I shook out my thoughts, I knew better than to forget that these patients were more normal than their stereotypes portrayed.

Returning her smile to hide my internal scolding, I asked if she would like to talk in her room. She agreed; she knew I was coming. She led me to her room and revealed its two unmade beds and two desks with litterings of wrappers and Styrofoam cups. I invited her to sit anywhere as we crossed the threshold and I shut the door. I felt like an intruder. She seemed like one, too, almost.

She chose to sit on her bed as I pulled out the incredibly heavy stool at the desk. She gently reminded that all the furniture was weighted for security. We both gave grimacing smiles at the reminder of just where we were… this was not two strangers chatting in the check-out line.

I introduced myself, trying to portray that I was just some ordinary student and not one of those ever studying (judging) psychiatrists.

Irrationally, I wanted her to believe I was just of those regular, relatable people that she could see out shopping for dish soap and milk. I laid my assignment on the table, I was here to interview her to find out how she got to the inpatient psych-ward for suicidal ideation. I reassured that this was her story, she could tell whatever she liked.

She started with the past couple years, but I discovered a lifetime of trauma and abuse. Her mother was a manipulative, neglectful narcissist that instilled issues that have lasted into adulthood. A cycle of self-esteem difficulties have led to multiple abusive romantic relationships. She has faced many manners of verbal, emotional, and physical abuse that ranged from beatings that required surgery to being forced to give up her new-born for adoption at the age of 18. My stomach sank as I continued to listen, she admitted to struggling with escaping domestic violence and suicidal ideation several times.

I asked why this time was different. Why did she escape this time after five years in the most recent relationship? She said that her young son tried to intervene on one of the beatings. Her children had witnessed mostly just screaming matches before. I hid another grimace. I asked why she sought help now. She wanted her children to have a mother and she planned on spending more time outdoors with them after treatment.

Internally, I prayed she stuck with it—for the kids at least. Aloud, I asked if I could tell her story of how ordinary people, even the most seemingly normal, can be subjected to cycles of abuse and that it is possible to escape.

STIGMA
SYDNEY SHOULDERS (CRS JULY 2023)

"Treat everyone how you want to be treated." This was the piece of advice that I was given by a cardiology patient that was a retired nurse. She was a geriatric nurse in a small town but had experience in many other settings, such as a jail, hospital, and rehab center. Although her heart was in geri-atrics, she said her favorite position was in the jail. When asked about the stigma that the inmates were rough, she said that the inmates themselves were not rough but that they were treated roughly by the policemen. She stated that you never know what someone has been through and described a horrific crime committed by the "most respectful man ever." She described to me her busy home life, as she lives with nine other people and her Chihuahua. She had two daughters and one son, but sadly she said that one of her daughters was killed in 2008. She grew up in a nearby town with her parents, two brothers, and one sister, and they were all very family oriented. One of the fondest memories of her childhood was sitting around the table and playing games with her family. As she grew up, she decided to become a Licensed Practical Nurse (LPN) and got her certification at the community college. She recently was in the hospital due to having atrial fibrillation for years that could not be shocked back into rhythm, so she had an ablation procedure. She also has a fairly new prosthetic leg that caused her to have phantom limb pain in the ankle region. She stated that for years she had patients describe this pain and she assumed that they just wanted a pain pill, but that her perspective has changed since becoming an amputee. I already hold the patient's piece of advice very close to my heart and plan to continue to do so as I move throughout my journey of becoming a physician.

UNSEEN BATTLE
SHAINA MAGNESS (PRE-CLINICAL JULY 2023)

When I asked the patient if I could ask him some questions and write about him, he enthusiastically told me that I had asked the right person. I asked him where he wanted to start, and he shook my hand as we exchanged names. He was 34, but he didn't tell me that until after he had me guess at his age, to which I had guessed 26. He was from our small town, had lived here his whole life. He grew up with his parents and seven siblings, which he was the second youngest of. In high school he was an athlete. Baseball, basketball, football, you name it, and it seemed he had played it. He went to college for computer science and technology, but sports were where he was most interested. Now he coaches little leagues and middle schools, his teams even winning several championships during his time as coach. He says he would love to go back to school so he could coach at colleges, but he thinks it is a little crazy that couching at that level requires a college degree despite his years of personal experience. When he is not coaching, he loves to go fishing. "I'll fish anywhere, I'm about to have to throw a line down one of these drains in here," he explained. When I asked him who he shared his home with he told me about his three girlfriends, three kids, and three dogs. He and two girlfriends lived together, while the third lived with three kids of her own. He said he recently had to drop down to just one girlfriend, because he suspected the others weren't being loyal. He said he is involved in his three children's lives, even when his teenage daughter might prefer that he not be quite so present, as teenagers are apt to do. Afterwards I asked if there was anything else I should know about him, to which he replied that he is the one and only, and after our conversation, I must agree that I haven't met someone quite like him before.

When I asked him what he thought I could do to be a good doctor, he turned it around and asked what I thought I should do to be a good doctor. I told him doing interviews like these are designed to help me learn to really listen to patients and that I think that is one of the greatest things a doctor can do. He added that one-on-one connection, confidentiality, and honesty are the things he likes most in a doctor. Having already attempted the first, I assured him that this paper would not include his name nor identification and that he could be provided with a copy if he likes.

The patient seemed like such a happy, funny, extroverted guy. Not someone who I would expect to see in the psych ward with a chart labeled "suicidal ideation," but rather someone I would expect to see cheering from the sidelines of a little league game. My conversation with him really reinforced the reality that mental health can be an unseen battle, waged internally amongst anyone in the community, such as a son, a student, a coach, a fisherman, or a patient.

CHAPTER 2

Learning to Relish Life from Working with My Patients

WHO REALLY WANTS TO BE SOMEONE'S DOCTOR? BILL CRUMP, M.D

For almost 40 years at four academic institutions, I took it as my personal mission to try to convince the right medical students to become family physicians. Policy experts say that we need to double or perhaps triple the number of graduating medical students that choose our specialty. There are tremendous barriers. We are not paid enough for our work as we co-ordinate our patients' care and the bureaucracy of prior authorizations and the tyranny of electronic medical records make it hard to get through the day with joy. But it is when the exam room door is closed and we can focus on the patient with us that we find that joy. Medical students are naturally risk-averse, and like to keep all of their options open. Many who are family doctors at heart choose Med-Peds just because they can keep the option open to subspecialize later and have a much easier life.

I asked Sarah Parker to put her thoughts on paper as she begins residency interviews as an example of a success. I first met her in 2015 when she did our college rural scholar program. Then she participated in our three-year accelerated medical school program that put her into a rigorous outpatient clerkship in the summer between her M-1 and M-2 years. In her M-3 year, she was clearly in her element when managing her continuity patients in our free clinic.

Sarah's essay reminds us all that no matter how busy we are, we can try to find the time to accommodate students in our practice. And it is just as important that they see us outside of the office advocating for our community. We must be doing something right.

SARAH PARKER (MS 4 MAY 2022)

Committing to a specialty is no easy task. After a single year of clinical training that is largely in the hospital, when you're finally getting comfortable, you must decide which direction to take for the rest of your career. Though I'd shadowed plenty of physicians in outpatient offices throughout college, I had next to no idea what went on in a hospital and I couldn't even dream up all the different services they have to offer. Growing up in Western Kentucky in my mom's beauty salon and dad's auto repair shop, I knew absolutely nothing about the differences among the ED, urgent care, or a primary care office. I quickly realized in medical school that what I enjoyed most was figuring out ways to get my patients the care they needed as easily and conveniently as possible and doing all of this so they wouldn't require hospitalization.

Because I wanted an even closer look at what it would be like to be a small town family doctor, I signed up to a complete clinical rotations for an accelerated track over the summer between my first and second year of medical school. This was my first true hands-on medical experience. I was handed a laptop and was set free to see basically everything that walked through the door. Here I learned what a full-spectrum doctor really looked like in action. After rounding on his hospital patients in the morning, my attending and I spent days seeing everything from Rocky Mountain spotted fever to brown recluse bites, bullous pemphigoid, and bilateral toenail removals. Here I saw the hodge-podge of medicine that healed each patient holistically, not just based on body system or condition. I really fell in love with being on the "front line" too. Every patient was like a mystery box.

Going into my 3rd year, I still didn't know with 100% certainty that family medicine was my calling. I knew I loved the outpatient primary care world, but the hospital was still a foreign place and along with it all those specialties that are primarily at the hospital: surgery, OB, internal medicine. I put these rotations first in my M-3 sequence. One by one, I found that I cared more about how they work together than how each one individually acted alone. EKGs are great, but the Cath lab is cold and dull. And how could I say goodbye to that cute kid after their appendix removal? I found myself collecting people. My favorite part was getting them ready for discharge. I loved being the one to sit down with my hand-written instructions on how to continue the healing process from home. I took care of some continuity patients at our student-directed free clinic. I cared for one uninsured patient with poorly controlled diabetes who made a strong impression. Over the course of a year, I helped manage a few medications through free drug manufacturer-sponsored patient assistance programs and lowered her Hemoglobin A1c from 11.5% to 7.1%. Coordinating all of this involved many lengthy conversations with my patient and I enjoyed the relationship I built with her over the course of a year. That's when I really knew family medicine was for me.

In addition, I realized early on that becoming a doctor, with all its hardships, would take me to a much higher socioeconomic level than I had when I was growing up. All the while, I would know that those working in the community alongside me provide services just as important and receive much lower compensation. I've always wanted to find ways to give back to my community outside of traditional medical care. In looking for that inspiration, everywhere I looked it seemed that family doctors were leading these endeavors. They run free clinics, nursing homes, health departments, addiction treatment centers, and attend local sports games. They are virtually everywhere the patients are and those qualities spoke to the heart and soul of why I chose to do medicine. This inspired me to create my own research project to interview our student-directed free clinic patients about their social determinants of health needs as part of an AAFP-sponsored leadership project.

I must say that the choice didn't come without some long hard talks with myself about why I even decided to become a doctor in the first place. Along the way, I met physicians I respected in other specialties that look down on family medicine physicians. In the end, I knew I was trading some super-specialized care for the training that would make me more versatile overall so I could attend to the needs of an entire person and entire communities. I knew that if I chose internal medicine, I'd be closing the door on a whole lot of training in outpatient care that I liked much more. I knew I'd be missing out on the huge amount of medicine that happens outside the hospital that I feel is even more important. I knew I couldn't be happy as a sub-specialist as I was already bored with seeing the same 5-6 diagnoses over and over again. I want to be as versatile as possible. I want to be trained in behavioral & addiction medicine, skin biopsies, LARCS and Pap smears, and have strong training in treatment of musculoskeletal injuries. When it comes to primary care, I knew that this versatility was incredibly important to my training and ultimately led me to choose family medicine.

20 YEARS FRESH
MICAH KAISER (MS 3 OCTOBER 2023)

Mr. Fred (not his real name) is a 43 year-old gentleman who was admitted to the Behavioral Health Unit for alcohol intoxication and suicidal ideation. He stated that he had been "clean" two times previously, once for 6 years and another time for 11 years; and that he ultimately wanted to try rehab again. He stated this episode of binge drinking had only lasted a couple weeks; unfortunately, he had severe withdrawals and had to be transferred to the Critical Care Unit. While speaking with him one day in the CCU and probing his suicidal ideation, he opened up to me. He said that he began drinking over 20 years ago after his young daughter, Ellie, had died in a car accident. One that had been entirely his fault. He explained that he and his spouse at the time were fighting vehemently in the car while she drove them home one rainy night—escalating to yelling, screaming, and her slapping his chest. He responded instinctively by trying to grab the steering wheel to pull the car off to the side of the road. His wife lost control and they spun into an oncoming 18-wheeler—killing his Ellie. His marriage broke down shortly after that, as did he.

As Mr. Fred told me the story, tears welled up in his eyes that ultimately led to wracking sobs. The pain and grief was as fresh today as it was 20 years ago. He still could not come to grips with the vast and shattering guilt from being responsible for the death of his daughter. It haunted him. Anytime he felt happiness, it would immediately be swallowed by a feeling of guilt due to his daughter not being alive due to his actions. He felt unworthy of joy; in a sense, he felt irredeemable. And so he punished and numbed himself with alcohol. Even as he was about to return to rehab he expressed that he was unsure if he would maintain his sobriety. He had done an unforgiveable act, one that he could not move on from nor accept. Ultimately, he was in the hospital for 2-weeks, and I spent a lot of time speaking and listening to him. At the time of his discharge, I shook his hand, wished him the best, and wondered if he would one day return again; still plagued by his inescapable regret.

Throughout my numerous encounters with Mr. Fred, I was continually struck by the gravity of how one moment had fractured this man's entire life. Not only that, but it had essentially frozen him in time. He was utterly unable to move past the moment his daughter died 20 years ago, his life remained mired in that one unforgiveable act. And I realized that he never would move on, not until he figured out how to accept it. To be honest, I am not sure that he will ever come to acceptance—he has spent the majority of his life carrying a weight that he feels he utterly deserves.

The encounter caused to me to be introspective about how much regret sometimes plays a role in my life. As medical students, we are used to holding ourselves to very high standards, and beating ourselves up when we don't reach them. However, this gentleman taught me first-hand how paralyzing regret can be, and how little I should let it take hold in my own life. I remember the intense sadness I continually felt in talking to Mr. Fred. He was a nice guy, but he had never experienced any growth or moved forward past this moment. He taught me that regretting the past can sometimes prevent you from improving the future.

Mr. Fred taught me several things that will make me a better physician. One is empathy for every patient I meet. Everyone has a story and a reason for the way they ended up, and trying to understand that story is critical to being a good healer. Second, live life forward, not backwards. It is incredibly easy to be frustrated and be mired down by "what-ifs"; however, being fixated on the past doesn't allow for future growth unless you accept and learn from your mistakes.

Being a good physician should be a process of continual growth. Lastly, I gained greater appreciation and gratitude for all the opportunities I have been afforded. It is truly a privilege to study medicine and to be able to have these meaningful encounters with patients, it is not a privilege I feel that I should take lightly.

A SINGING LADY WITH A SERVANT'S HEART
MARIA SHIELDS (PRE-MATRIC JUNE 2020)

One of Ms. M's earliest memories was getting her tonsils and adenoids taken out at the age of 5. Her dad promised her a dog if she cooperated - a Cocker Spaniel to be exact. For days after the procedure, popsicles became her new best friend. Soon after, she wedged her fingernail in the door of a station wagon. Other than this minor injury and surgical procedure, Ms. M recalls that she was a healthy child. Ms. M married her husband at the age of 19 and had her first child at the age of 24 followed by her son. She also has an adopted son giving her a total of 3 children. From her children, she has many grandchildren ranging in age from 5 to 28.

Ms. M's father was a seminary pastor who lectured at the local church. Ms. M's mother passed away from thyroid cancer when she was a young girl. She recalls when her mother first starting suffering from the feeling a pressure "sitting on her neck". After further examination, it was found that her T4 hormone levels were elevated and cancer was later diagnosed. As a result of her mother's progressively worsening health, Ms. M often did a lot of the cooking in the home as a child. At the age of 7, Ms. M sat at the edge of the bed where her mother lay ill and learned how to make homemade bread.

When they were growing up in Portland, she mentions that they lived in close proximity to the Columbia River where toxic waste was often dumped from upstream nuclear power plants. In the 1900s, the U.S. Department of Energy built nine nuclear reactors along the Columbia River to produce plutonium and other radioactive materials. A site in Hanford released approximately 725,000 curies of radioactive iodine-131 between the years of 1944 and 1957. Long-term exposure to radioactive iodine-129 has been found to cause thyroid cancer while low doses prevents proper function in the thyroid gland. To the horror of the public, large air-borne releases of radioactive iodine from Hanford have been blamed for decades of thyroid illnesses in surrounding communities. Included in this morbidity, are Ms. M and her brother who have both been diagnosed with Hashimoto's thyroiditis. She struggles with the secondary side effects of this, as well as arthritis, high blood pressure, and some gastrointestinal problems. With great sadness, I reflected upon

the great influence of how someone's place of birth often inevitably affects their overall health outcomes and conditions. I was distressed at the
thought of Ms. M's siblings and mother suffering from the effects of their
once toxic home.

Ms. M has fond memories from her time as a world-traveling singer at
the age of 25. She remembers getting her first physical examination at
the age of 17 so that she could spend nearly 4 weeks traveling Europe to
sing and raise money for cancer research. She even remembers singing
for the Lord Mayor of London. Ms. M's love for traveling didn't stop as
a young girl, however. Today, she has the accolade of visiting every U.S.
state (excluding Alaska). She has also held onto her love of singing and
music and now plays piano at her church as a part of their praise and
worship services. She also occasionally traveled to France and Germany
to visit her son who was a member of the U.S. Navy. I got the impression
that these were some of the best moments of Ms. M's life - her eyes lit up
with excitement.

As I was talking to Ms. M, I couldn't help but be reminded of Disney's
princess Belle. Belle loves to read about all kinds of people and places in
her library and her understanding of these unknown people and destina-
tions enables her to open her heart to love those that others rarely see
value in. Similar to Belle, Ms. M's love for knowledge and appreciation
for all people is reflected in her volunteerism and care for both her students and nursing home residents alike. Ms. M takes on diverse identities
and roles in the lives of her loved ones; she is truly a jack-of-all trades.
To her grandchildren, she is the creator of "Yahoo Punch" - a delicious
concoction of Fruit Punch and Jell-O. To her nursing home residents, she
is the singing lady - a source of joy and happiness. To her students, she is
the beloved favorite substitute teacher among many. Ms. M has a servant's
heart that seeks to bring joy to the lives of those around her. When she
sees a need, she fills it. Ms. M's life aligns precisely to what she considers
to her life motto of J.O.Y. - Jesus, Others, and You. She is a firm believer
in giving to others simply out of pure love and kindness.

A WOMAN WHO UNDERSTANDS THE IMPORTANCE OF PERSPECTIVE
SUMMER SPARKS (CRS JULY 2020)

Attitude is everything. It is amazing how a positive attitude can directly produce a positive outcome. Mrs. X, a patient who is now in her early 60's can testify to the importance of optimism and how her ability to see good in even the most hopeless situation has dramatically affected her life for the better.

She began her story by describing her picturesque childhood which she shared with loving and present parents along with 6 siblings. Being the oldest girl child, she developed an independent streak early in her life. She also inferred that she was insatiably curious. As a young child, she had seen her parents and grandparents smoking cigarettes and she wanted to give it a try. She jovially depicted how when she struck a match to light a cigarette, she accidently caught her flannel night gown on fire, and she showed me the scars to prove it! Mrs. X also wanted to emphasize that her fondest early memories involved spending time with those she loved most. She enjoyed riding around her hometown with her father and siblings in her family's red convertible. In another anecdote, she told me how fortunate she was to be able to walk only three houses down to her grandparent's house where her grandmother would let her pin-curl her hair.

As a young adult, Mrs. X found herself far from her small Kentucky home. She moved to a suburb of Manhattan when she was only 20 years old. As aforementioned, she had an investigative mind and craved new experiences. She also said that over time, she developed a drinking habit, and her life became centered on partying. This habitual drinking eventually led to a strained relationship with her present husband. She was not proud of the person she had become, but the habit continued, nonetheless.

Unfortunately, on a rainy October night in 1987, she made a life chang-ing decision. She rode home from a party with a friend who had also been drinking that night. As the two friends drove down the seemingly deserted road, Mrs. X became nervous about her friend's driving competency. She urged her friend to let her drive. The friend relinquished her duty as driver and pulled over. As Mrs. X walked around the car to the driver's side, another driver drove speedily down the road. The driver had a defect in her bumper where a sharp edge jutted out horizontally. Mrs. was so disoriented from being intoxicated that she was having difficulty opening the door to her car. As the driver closely passed the girls' parked car, Mrs. X's left leg was caught by the driver's deformed bumper. The driver unknowingly dragged Mrs. 48 feet (more than half the length of an Olympic-sized swimming pool) before noticing her.

Mrs. X went on to tell me that she does not remember much about the incident and only remembers waking up in the hospital a few days later. Mrs. X had to be resuscitated twice that night and lost half of her leg. She was later informed that she would never walk again and, most devastating to Mrs. X, that she would never bear children.

Mrs. X then strangely began to smile. She explained that although it was a terrible accident, she was glad that it had happened to her. She perceived the incident as a "wake-up call" from God. She believed that it was God's way of asking her to change her lifestyle and to stop being self-destructive. From that point onward, Mrs.'s life changed. Her life became about serving others and having gratitude. With this radiant positivity, she defied all odds. She eventually regained the ability to walk and a few years later gave birth to her daughter.

Today, Mrs. X is living her dream. She pursues her passion for art and sewing, and even is a part-time DJ. She is also looking forward to being a grandmother. I asked her what advice she had for me as a young person and aspiring physician. She told me to always believe that good things can happen. She also told me to always have sympathy for others without pitying them. I was incredibly blessed to hear Mrs. X's story, and I will not forget her wise advice.

It is so easy to focus on all the negativity in the world, but the truth is, there is just as much good if one is looking for it. Mrs. X was involved in a tragic event, and yet she did not want pity. It is human nature to feel sorry for individuals who have experienced difficult life circumstances, however, many of those individuals are proud that they have had the fortitude to overcome such challenges.

I also think that it is interesting how many patients who refuse to be defeated by their afflictions often have better health outcomes. I had never realized exactly how important a patient's attitude and faith affected his or her physical well-being. As a result, I want to spread hope to my patients and uplift their spirits when they seem dejected. This may, in fact, be just as important as providing medications to alleviate their aliments.

Lastly, I want to learn from Mrs. X's example. I hope to be a person who is optimistic and brave like she is. Anyone can have a positive attitude when his or her life is going well, but it takes true courage to stay positive in the midst of a trying life-event.

BEER OLYMPICS IN ROOM 4
EMILY BOLINGER (CRS JULY 2020)

As soon as the day started, the doctor I was shadowing was trying to help me find someone to interview. As he scrolled through his schedule for the day, he contemplated a few patients. "I found you one. Go in room 4. She's a hoot," he said with a chuckle. I went in and greeted her. I explained that I was with the University of Louisville School of Medicine Trover campus for the summer, and we are doing patient interviews. She was nodding as I went on to say that these are not interviews about your health status, but I want to hear about your life outside of being a patient. She was cordial and seemed willing to talk. She said she is 70 years old and she grew up close to here. She was a local and has been all her life. She said she was divorced, but they had twins: a boy and a girl. One lived in Louisville and the other lives close by. She reminisced as she told me about her little brother. "He was thirteen years younger than me, and I swear he was on my hips more than his own mother's," she laughed and expressed that she basically raised him. Today, they are still as close as they were back then. From what I can tell, this woman is the jack of all trades. "I have done a little bit of everything, you know. I was a teacher then I was a business-woman, and I also ran a restaurant," she said with pride. Now she is retired. She spends her days at her lakeside home reading and drinking beer. "You can't live at the lake and not drink beer," she said with humor after I asked her how she spends her retirement. She has three grandkids. As we wrapped up, I wondered if she was happy with her life how it is. She expressed that she was very pleased with her life. "My friends are a lot younger than me. They like me because I can keep up with them," she said while we both laughed together. I told her that I don't doubt that she would be right there with them. She said she loves her kids and grandkids because they have a lot of the same interests as her. Her advice to me as a future doctor was simple. "You have a good personality. Don't change that. That's important to make your patients feel comfortable, so they will talk to you," she said as she encouraged me to stick with it and work hard. The doctor walked in as we had just finished. Further into the visit he asked, "Are you having the beer Olympics this year?" She laughed and said she did not know due to the pandemic at hand. She explained to me how she holds the beer Olympics every year at the lake, and she usually wins. We shared a long laugh while she told the doctor she expects him to be there if she hosts it again. We exited and had a laugh when we got back to the doc's office.

I am so glad my doctor sent me to room 4 this week. It is such a reset to encounter someone who doesn't take life too seriously. Yes, I am sure the retirement has something to do with her lack of worries, but I feel she has always been young at heart. As a potential medical school student, meeting her has been nothing short of luck. The day to day can really get you down. There is a lot of mental pressure when preparing for medical school: constant studying, pressure to do more, comparing yourself to others, and competitive peers. It is easy to get so caught up on to-do lists that I forget it's okay to relax for a while and laugh. After I left the interview, I immediately felt a little bit of relief from my anxieties. I felt like I had gained a perspective: that life can be fun even in the struggle. Obviously, this woman has had hardships with a divorce and some hard jobs, but all the while she maintained her young spirit. She is content. And I think we can all be content if we look past the serious and take a little pressure off of ourselves. So, the next time I get too caught up in the stress of life, I am going to remember that it is okay to "drink a beer by the lake" sometimes.

HARD COPY OF HISTORY
IAN LEATHERMAN (CRS JULY 2021)

Patient gives Dr. Z a stapled sheet of paper of daily things she thinks is wrong with her health.

"You are wasting your energy on negativity; you will have no energy for positivity."

Listen to your body and don't fall into the compulsivity of writing about your health. "Come out of it."

Worry about living your life, not documenting it.

LOVE ALL AROUND
SARAH FISHER (MS 3 OCTOBER 2014)

Most of all, my patients have taught me about love – loving life, loving each other, and loving yourself. I watched one of my patients fight for every minute of his life, despite an aggressive cancer, and I watched his wife fight even harder. One of my patients from our free clinic brings his wife to every visit, and she is so dedicated to his health that she has changed both of their diets to help him. While in the hospital, I witnessed a woman who chose to love herself and carry on, even after her husband left her. All of these acts of love have deeply inspired me to love even greater. I am more purposeful about enjoying life, especially outside of medicine. I love on my family, and appreciate my friendships daily. Not only that, but I began to love myself and celebrate all I have to offer others.

Some of my greatest teachers have been my patients. They have imparted lessons of appreciation, love, acceptance, and joy during my short time with them. My patients also have taught me other lessons that are imprinted on my heart: everyone deserves a good hairstyle; a sip of Dr. Pepper is sometimes the best taste in the world; and that loneliness is the worst illness of all. My patients, my teachers: these individuals are the unsung heroes of medical education.

LOVING LIFE
SUMMER SPARKS (CRS JULY 2020)

Mr. G is 64 years old and is, according to his primary care physician, in fantastic health. He told me that he stays in such great shape because his is so active. He was born in Kentucky and has lived there for much of his life. He and his wife currently live in Western Kentucky. He began by telling me that when he was younger, he loved to play with his older brother. They would go to ball games and fish at a nearby pond. He said he did this until his brother was sixteen and was able to drive. His brother was then "too cool" to hang out with his little brother. He loved to swim, and his parents had a swimming pool at their residence. He was close to his parents, but they worked a lot. He said that his parents owned a nursing home that was near to where they lived. I also asked if he liked school. He said that he absolutely loved school and that he was always good at it. He seemed to excel at history and science.

After high school, he attended the University of Kentucky. There, he received a bachelor's degree in Business Management. Soon after he graduated, he moved back to his hometown to work at his family's nursing home. He soon married one of his childhood friends. She, too, worked at the nursing home as an RN. They still live in the first house they bought together as a young couple.

A few years later they had two sons. The boys grew up playing many sports which Mr. G helped coach. Today, they are still a close family and Mr. G has two granddaughters. He loves watching them play in the community youth soccer league. Mr. G is now retired and has many hobbies. One of his favorite things to do is to travel to new places. His favorite vacation destination is the Cayman Islands. He says that he enjoys anything outside. He enjoys taking walks with his Labrador retriever. He has a thriving garden where he grows many vegetables including squash and tomatoes. His favorite activity, however, is cycling. He competes in bike races, and he also loves to mountain bike. He had a knee injury several years ago, and claims he has a little arthritis. His knee still bothers him while cycling. He hopes to improve this issue in order to continue to do what he loves. He says that other than his knee issue, he is "loving life".

This patient exhibited great joy for living. He seemed like he really enjoyed spending time with his friends and family. The advice that he wanted to give me as a future physician is to always be honest and do the right thing even when it is difficult. He also was very encouraging and told me to never give up on my dream of become a physician. I hope to follow his example as I grow older. I want to take care of myself so that I am still able to partake in activities that I love even when I'm a little older. He also never lets his bad knee dampen his spirits, and he always gives his best during races even when he is in pain. He also reminds me of why I really want to go into a medical profession. I want to improve others' qualities of life. With treatment, he will be able to find his activities more enjoyable because he will be in far less pain.

OLD MACDONALD HAD A FARM
CIERRA WOODCOCK (CRS JULY 2020)

Mrs. MacDonald (not her real name) is 60 -year- old woman that grew up in the heart of Western Kentucky. She came in the office complaining of severe back pain. According to her, it was getting worse and she could no longer work on the farm the way she used to. It was so bad that day, she could barely walk and was forced to use a wheelchair.

Mrs. M was the epitome of southern hospitality, with her kind personality and outgoing sense of humor. After informing the doctor that she had grown up on a farm and lived on one her whole life, it was easy to see that being a farmer was something she was truly passionate about. She even cracked the joke that she was "old M that had a farm." She told stories about growing vegetables to hand out to locals, riding horses, camping, and all of her exotic pets that she had over the years. She then began to talk about how she used her farm to help her community and to bring joy to those around her. The most interesting story that Mrs. M told was about her wild turkey that she had tamed and all of the adventures they had been on together. She said that the turkey is just like any other pet, listening to commands and coming when called for. Mrs. M said that the turkey had been on many road trips with her and her husband, and that the turkey would just set around the campfire like a person. The best part about her having the turkey as a pet was when she mentioned that she took it to the local nursing home for all the residents to see. She laughed saying, "it was the most wonderful thing I've ever done. The residents loved him as he strutted down the hall, gobbling when they touched him. The turkey loved it too, he really thought he was a hot shot getting all of that attention from those elderly people." Seeing how passionate Mrs. M was about her farm and her pets, made it easy to understand why she wanted to get rid of her back pain. The doctor mentioned that she had "the spine of a hard worker," meaning that in the X-Ray it was slightly crooked. He said it was due to all of her hard work on the farm over the years. He told her that he could send her to a pain clinic to manage the pain and she would be back to working on the farm in no time. Her eyes lit up like the lights on a Christmas tree. She could finally get back to doing what she loved the most.

This patient really stood out to me because I know what it is like to grow up on a farm and I enjoyed every second of it the way that she had. I also knew how it made her feel when she could not work on her farm because she was in so much pain. It made me realize that I will not always be as fit as I am now, and I should be more considerate of the older population because they were once young like me. The doctor said that he could have suggested back surgery to fix her problem, but it was likely she would never be able to do the kind of work she does now, especially at her age. As a future physician, it made me want to work harder to preserve the quality of life in my patients, not just fix the problem and the patient never be able to return to what they love. It is not always about curing every ailment, sometimes it is just about doing what is best for the patient to be happy. Life is not worth living if you cannot live it doing what you love.

OUT IN THE ELEMENTS
DREW DODDS (PRE-CLINICAL JULY 2022)

Patient D is a mid-50s male who was born and raised in Western Kentucky. He has a 23 year old son who is a hardworking man! He is currently married and can't wait to give his wife a big kiss when he is discharged from the hospital. Growing up, he had a large number of pets including his favorite dog, a 6 foot boa snake, and several horses just to name a few. He loved to fish, party and have family get-togethers growing up. He had an elder brother and sister who have passed but still has a younger brother alive. His mom worked at the locally famous doughnut shop when he was growing up.

Patient D decided to stop school in 6th grade and decided to work on a horse farm where he was able to keep several famous individuals' horses. In school though, his favorite subjects were science, math and history. He has also worked for a saw mill making power line poles and was actually working in when there were 4 major hurricanes and the locally destructive tornado in the fall of 2005. Patient D was working that fall day when the tornado came through and remembers hearing it as well as taking cover. His family's luck with tornadoes hasn't proven great unfortunately because in the record breaking long distance tornado that destroyed part of Western Kentucky in December of 2021, his nephew's wife's grandparents had their house destroyed.

Patient D presented with kidney stones and after a few days in the hospital, can't wait to get home to his wife. His favorite food he is looking forward to eating is meatloaf and mashed potatoes but all breakfast food is a close second and might even be the next meal. He thinks his best future is a little bit of a healthier lifestyle after taking better care of his health.

Lastly, Patient D thinks the best thing medical students can be taught is how to talk, connect and just listen to patients. He thinks listening to patients will significantly improve the patient physician relationship and is hopeful the next generation of doctors will connect with patients more than some doctors he has had previously.

PRAYING FOR UNLIMITED MOBILITY
SUMMER SPARKS (PRE-CLINICAL JULY 2022)

Ms. ES was born in Indiana in 1938. At age 2, her mother passed away, and she was inherited and raised by her aunt. Ms. ES has a brother and a sister still living. She also had two older brothers who died before she was born. She completed her education up to 8th grade. After leaving school, she began her career at the local GE plant. At the plant, her responsibilities included cleaning the plant and some machinery. Soon after that, she met and married her wonderful husband. She currently lives in Western Kentucky, where she's lived for 50 years. Later on, she was also employed by several banks where she was responsible for housekeeping. She is very proud of her family, and her family is a very important part of her life. She spends a lot of time with them because many of them live near her. She has three children currently. She, unfortunately, lost a child when he was very young. Understandably, this was a very difficult experience for Ms. ES. Ms. ES is also proud of the fact that she is a grandmother and also a great-grandmother. She is an active participant in many groups at her church. Her favorite hobby is reading. She explained that she loves to read so much that she was willing to read any reading material regardless of its content. When asked her favorite things to read specifically she said, "Her bible". She also said that she enjoys reading magazines and news articles. She stated, "She loves staying up to date on what is going on in the world".

Ms. ES feels as if she really needs to get her back pain under control. She is often frustrated by the fact that she is not as mobile anymore. Her children often worry that she will fall if she has to walk far distances. She understands this, but because of her reduced mobility, she can no longer do many things that she used to enjoy, such as spending time outdoors. Ms. ES believes that her best immediate future will include being discharged from the hospital where she can go back to her home. She is excited about relaxing in her comfortable chair and playing with her fox terrier. In her best long-term future, she hopes that her health will improve so that she can travel again. Her favorite place to travel is California. Her best advice for an upcoming physician is to always work hard and give 100% effort.

THE ARTIST
KENNEDY BREEDING (PRE-MATRIC JUNE 2020)

Mrs. H is an 83-year-old female who loves to spend her free time coloring. She was born and raised in a small town with 4 siblings. Mrs. H describes her childhood as not the best but certainly not the worst either. "We had everything we needed and some of the things we wanted", she explains as she rhythmically folded her handkerchief in her hands.

After getting her degree in accounting, Mrs. H and her engineer husband settled in another town where they worked for the same company. They stayed there for 22 years until her husband began having heart problems. They then moved to a neighboring county where they farmed and raised horses. During her time here, she used her spare time to make dolls for local children while her husband made doll sized love seats to accompany them. Her favorite being a humpty dumpty set. She describes gingerly setting the 20 inch dolls on the love seat that her husband had crafted. I always put Mr. Humpty's arm around Mrs. Humpty and they just looked so cute!"

Mrs. H has a love for children, particularly her own. She beams with pride and displays a smile that seems to stretch across her entire face and radiates throughout her body every time she mentions her son. "I had the most wonderful son that ever lived", she explained. She went on to tell stories of her son helping other kids with homework, going back to school to become a local high school teacher and always spending time with her and her husband.

Then the smile slowly began to lose its brilliance as she entered the next part of her tale. She began explaining how her son spent even more time with her after her husband died. However, it was only a few months following that event that he was diagnosed with advanced cancer and only given one year to live.

Mrs. H spent the next thirteen months taking care of her son. Using her passion for cooking to cope with the stress, she made him everything he possibly wanted. "My homemade vegetable soup was the last thing he ate before going into the hospital", she recalled. Unfortunately that would be his last homemade meals as he passed away in the hospital shortly after.

Mrs. H then explained that she was not by his side. Her son had refused to let her go to the hospital for fear that she would get the flu. Because she had been so busy with him, she forgot to get the vaccine. Despite the painful experience of losing her son Mrs. H refuses to be negative, saying he's gone to a better place. "I have to look at it that way to get through", she revealed with a decided nod of her head.

Shortly after losing her son, Mrs. was admitted to the hospital for blood pressure problems. She was quickly released and sent to a neighboring mental health hospital to spend Christmas which was only a few days away and would be the first without her son. She then told a story of seeing a man at the hospital sitting alone coloring and explained that her son always recommended coloring as a way to stay occupied. So she picked up a colored pencil and began. She spent the next month coloring and was then discharged.

After her discharge she moved to an apartment where one of her few remaining family members, her nephew, checked in on her as well as a fellow apartment tenant whom she grew close to. She continued coloring from then on and says she sends them to nursing homes to bring others joy.

Presently Mrs. H finds herself in the hospital due to psychosis that appears in the form of voices in her head. Most recently, sing song voices that chant that she will die as she tries to sleep. Her face tenses with anxiety as she discusses her final night at her apartment before she decided enough was enough. Mrs. H says since coming to the hospital she feels much safer and the voices only come when she has extensive testing done but are not as threatening. They now chant about her blue jeans. "I don't blame them", she says with a chuckle, "I've had the same jeans for twenty years and they still look great on me."

Mrs. H says she is content with her life and likes the facilities because they give her ample time to color, the thing her son wanted her to do. In fact, as I asked if she was willing to do an interview she was working on a picture of an elephant that was being shaded with bright shades of fuchsia. "It's been a good life", she explains as we finish the interview and I return her to her coloring station. Mrs. H smiled as she looked at the arsenal of colored pencils, sharpened and at the ready for her to finish her elephant.

THE FRIEND SAYING FAREWELL
KENNEDY BREEDING (PRE-MATRIC JUNE 2020)

When I started my day in the psychiatric unit in the hospital, I was greeted with a "Yippee." The exclamation came from an elderly woman resting in a wheelchair in-between the entrance and the nurse's station. She was dressed in a powder blue night gown with matching sweater and displayed a huge smile across her face. When I made my way to the nurse's station, one of the on-duty nurses told me that that was Mrs. C., who just found out she was getting discharged later that day.

As the day passed, Mrs. C buzzed excitedly throughout the geriatric side of the unit. When I asked her for a quick interview, she readily agreed and began telling me about herself.

Mrs. was born and raised in Nashville Tennessee. She explained that during her childhood Nashville was a far cry from the Country Music Capital it is today and it wasn't until after she married her high school sweetheart and moved away that it began to resemble the Nashville that we know. However, Mr. and Mrs. made many trips back to The Music City because they both shared a love of country music. Looking as if she could still hear the melody resonating in her ears, she began to spit out a large and very impressive list of acts that she had seen.

"Conway Twitty, Garth Brooks, Lauren Morgan. We've seen 'em all", she said with a nod of her head. "And kept all of my ticket stubs!" My ears perked up with familiarity at that last sentence. As an avid music fan myself, I keep all of my ticket stubs in a binder. As I explained that to her and she chuckled and said, "Yep, I just keep them in a big stack held together with a rubber band. It's nice to have them for memories." I shook my head in agreement, knowing exactly how she felt. Would I be 80 years old, flipping through the pages of my ticket binder, reliving the excitement of a large crowd, the buzz of amplifiers and the pure joy you get when your favorite act takes the stage?"

Mrs. C continued to talk about music for a while after that, musing over her favorite musician Alan Jackson and even disclosing a time when she left her ticket at home by mistake and sweet talked her way into the door.

Other than music, Mrs. C's other passion is boating. When Mr. and Mrs. C began to settle down and have a family, they invested in an RV and boat to use at a nearby lake during the warm months. Mr. C was an avid fisher, but Mrs. C made it clear that she wasn't too bad herself. "You should see the one that I caught and had mounted!"

Mrs. C and her family visited the lake for 25 years and made many memories with her children and grandchildren there. However, once Mr. C became too ill to fish, they gifted the boat to their son for him to continue building new memories with their grandson. Mrs. C said that she was still capable of fishing but couldn't stand the thought of leaving her husband at home to go.

Mrs. C called her husband from the hospital every morning to check in. As luck would have it, today, the very day she would get discharged, she had not. "I thought he may be sleeping and didn't want to bother him", she explained. Mr. C had kidney problems. When I asked what brought Mrs. C into the hospital she said that she couldn't remember. I later found out that it was due to late onset Alzheimer's and couldn't help but image the ailing Mrs. C trying her best to take care of Mr. C as her own health deteriorated. That's when we began discussing her departure.

She took a deep breath as if the thought hadn't crossed her mind before and said, "You know, I've been here for two or three weeks and you get attached to the people here." With that she nodded at the lady sitting next to her. She explained that the two have been in the unit for the same amount of time and was going to miss their daily conversations and debates over Jeopardy answers. "We're just like sisters now. Leaving is just going to get me right here", she said gesturing at her heart.

However, when I asked her what she was going to do when she got home, her excited smile returned. She pretended to recline in her wheelchair and prop up her feet and enthusiastically said, "Sit in my recliner and drink two cups of coffee!" She explained that the unit only had decaf which wasn't real coffee and she was more than ready to indulge in multiple cups of the stuff.

Soon after that, the wheelchair came for Mrs. C's transport and she hurriedly rushed to her room to put on a pair of clean clothes and wash her face. I stayed sitting with her friend who would soon be left alone. Noticeably sad, she said that she was glad to have met a lady like Mrs. C while in the hospital and only hoped whoever was filling her spot was just as nice. And just like that they loaded up Mrs. C and wheeled her out of the unit. As she waved at all of the patients and nurses, I heard a nurse sigh under her breathe "Sad to see her go. I'm going to miss her." It was clear that Mrs. C had been an intricate part of the ward's dynamic the last two weeks and had made friends with both the patients and staff.

THE IMPORTANCE OF FAMILY
CAITLAN JONES (CRS JULY 2020)

"To get my s*** together." This is what Cory (not his real name) wants. When asked at the end of the day what he wants after his treatment is completed, that was his immediate response. Cory is a lighthearted, funny 29-year-old who resides in Western Ky. Growing up Cory was the only boy with one step-sister and two biological sisters. Like all families, Cory's relationships with his sisters varied; he and his younger sister have always been thick as thieves while him and his older sister butted heads a lot. Although when life threw him a curve ball and he was down on his luck, it was his older sister who reached out to help. And they have been mending their relationship ever since. A father with two daughters of his own, Cory is now currently living with his older sister and explained that her children have become like his too. Trained in a variety of construction techniques and skills, his favorite is laying flooring. His sister's family owns a construction company that Cory recently worked for. However, he explained that finding a new job with different people, even in an entirely new industry is what he believes is best for his health. After a series of unfortunate events and feelings of hopelessness, Cory has found just how important his life is and many new ways to better take care of himself mentally. Finding people that he shares a common ground with that have gone through similar experiences that he has is what he said has helped the most. He also mentioned that he hoped I would get to meet Brad and Dr. A as they had been a great help and were really nice people. He said that the person I interviewed was who he really was that I would not have recognized him before he started treatment. He was beaming and smiling, eager to share his story and how great it felt to do a 180. When asked about what quality he wished all doctors had his answer was simple: a personality. He wants the facts and to be talked to directly, but also to feel heard and understood. That bedside manner is important. Cory shared that in high school he suffered a knee injury and went to the doctor asking for help. He said the doctor didn't believe him and aggressively bent and twisted his knee, only making the injury worse. He wanted help and to feel heard. While Cory may have not got that feeling nearly 15 years ago for an orthopedic injury, he does now. Cory is still finishing up treatment but is continually getting closer and closer to getting back on track and getting his s*** back together.

Cory was young, energetic, and very easy to talk too. Cory is currently a patient in the behavioral unit. To be honest, I was very nervous to shadow in Psychiatry. I was afraid I would have trouble connecting to patients and learning what was appropriate to say and what was not. However, my time shadowing made all those nerves go away, and talked with Cory about all things life was a big part of that. It's often easy to think that hurting people, sick people, or someone seeking mental health help are not "normal". However, I was quickly convicted that that assumption is not accurate. Cory was a county boy who loved his 5 dogs, kids, and sitting on the front porch. He had just hit a rough patch recently and needed help getting out of it. Dr. N, whom I shadowed, had talked a lot about the biopsychosocial model of health and illness. We often forget the importance of the social aspect, and Cory's telling of how it assisted with his healing was some real-life evidence. I realize that isolation is not the answer to improving one's health, instead human interactions can be key. It makes one curious as to how the increased isolation due to COVID-19 has affected the mental health of millions of people. It makes one question, how much hurt has months of isolation and missing the social aspect caused?

FAR FROM *DETH*
TARYN MIRACLE (PRE-MATRIC JUNE 2020)

Mr. G will be 83 years old in September. He is a resident of Western KY. Mr. G has high blood pressure and cholesterol but still feels "perfect." Last time he saw his doctor he had to double his blood pressure medication. He now takes two pills in the morning and one cholesterol pill at night. He keeps a blood pressure record but forgot to bring it with him. He remembered his blood pressure as 126/72 before leaving the house. He has had no issues since last June when he found out he had cancer.

Last year, Mr. G was told he had melanoma on his foot and needed to remove it as soon as possible. He went to the hospital where they ended up having to remove his big toe. He occasionally experiences swelling around the ankle that he believes is from the amputation. He also had a hip surgery where one of his legs was replaced with bone from his arm. He had no idea that could be done, but he is glad it did.

Mr. G is a father of six. He has one biological son, one biological daughter, and four children from his wife's previous marriage. Mr. G helped raised his wife's children, putting them through school. He and his wife did it together, but he takes great pride in having supported them and making sure they had everything they needed. He and his wife have been married 53 years. He says he spends his time taking care of his wife who also has cancer and heart problems. She has leukemia and requires a pill three times each day. He plans to leave the clinic, go home, and take care of his wife.

Mr. G has spent his life working. He started adulthood early by serving in the military for five years as a teenager. He spent nine years driving a truck after working in an oil field for nine years. He worked at York for the next seventeen years.

Mr. G keeps forgetting to bring his advanced directive to the clinic. He wants it scanned into their system so that there is record of it. He hand-wrote this document concerning his "deth." He has had a "pretty good life" and wants to make sure he cares for his family.

IT RUNS IN THE FAMILY
ELAINA PERRY (PRE-MATRIC JUNE 2022)

Patient X is a 49-year-old, Caucasian male born in Kentucky. Growing up he had three brothers and four sisters, two of which recently died of strokes. At the age of four, he and his family moved from Kentucky to Michigan where he spent most of his childhood. Patient X's parents were factory workers. Growing up, patient X spent time playing with his siblings. His family was very close. He also spent a lot of time in the garage with his father working on car engines. He learned decent mechanic skills that would later come in handy on small side jobs throughout his life. Patient X graduated from a high school in Michigan. After graduating, patient X worked in construction. He was also a painter. Along the way, patient X had a girlfriend with whom he had his first son. He later had his second son with another girlfriend. Both of his sons decided to follow in their father's footsteps, becoming painters. Patient X now has multiple grandchildren which he adores. About nine years ago, patient X moved back to Kentucky. He has most recently been working as a painter. He spends his free time fishing and hunting. While patient X does enjoy rifle hunting, he prefers to hunt with more primitive weapons like bow and muzzleloader because he believes that it is more "die hard". Patient X is currently recovering from a stroke which has left him with no motor function on the left side of his body. After recovery and release from the hospital, patient X hopes to spend as much time as possible with his sons and his grandchildren.

PRESENT DIFFICULTIES
KATELYN MATTINGLY (CRS JULY 2023)

Sometimes diagnoses can feel defining and depressing. It was obvious that for this patient, discussing her health was saddening for her. She has been battling COPD for 15 years and was diagnosed with heart failure this time. She was a kind person and enjoyed simple living. Her excitement that she got to go home that day showed. After some effort, I could see the patients' eyes light up when getting to talk about some of the things that make her who she is.

Before asking any questions, I could tell that her family meant a lot to her, and she to them. She received two phone calls from people checking in on her just in the hour that we were in the room. She later told us that she has 6 children, 3 boys and 3 girls. She was proud of them. They had all grown up, had children of their own, and some had moved to different states. Between her kids and siblings, she has family living in Texas, Georgia, Virginia and here in Kentucky. It always makes me sad when families move away from each other. I was glad to hear she still has family here and lives with her eldest son. Her son and his family take care of her. They cook her meals, help her get around and do daily tasks such as bathing.

It took a couple minutes for this patient to open up about her past. I can imagine that the present difficulties can make it easy to forget about the good times of the past. Especially since in the past 15 years there has been much that she has not been able to do. This patient grew up in a small town in Kentucky where she spent a lot of time working. Her need to make money hindered her from having perfect attendance at school, but she pushed through and was able to graduate. I could tell through our conversation that she was a hard worker for many years and overcame a lot of obstacles. I admire that. She worked at a factory for 35 years where she got to enjoy her passion for sewing blue jeans. She no longer sews, but I could tell she still loves the thought of it. I loved talking to her about the things she used to enjoy, but it saddened me that she feels she no longer can. Cooking is one of these things she used to enjoy as well. When I asked the patient what her favorite thing to cook was, she told me "Whatever the kids wanted", but everyone loved her banana pudding. Since moving in with her son, she doesn't cook much because she doesn't feel like she has her own space. This made me appreciate the importance of pursuing hobbies through old age. It gives a sense of identity that is necessary to survival. We should always remember we are allowed to take up space and make new memories.

CHAPTER 3

Lessons in Resilience

A DIFFERENT TYPE OF STRENGTH
SUMMER SPARKS (PSYCHIATRY ROTATION JULY 2023)

One of my first few days as a third-year medical student, I am still attempting to find my way around the hospital and understand my basic responsibilities. I was eager to learn much from my new attendings and to start helping patients solve problems. I had little exposure to psychiatry, except for shadowing here and there; however, I have found that many patients' stories are genuine, unfiltered, and often very sad. One patient I saw with my attending, Dr. A, had a story that was especially poignant.

James entered the exam room. He was around 6 feet tall and appeared burly and masculine. He explained that he worked as a delivery driver for many years and occasionally did manual labor jobs. It surprised me that a man who appeared this tough could be so sad. James explained to us why he was admitted to the inpatient psychiatric facility. He explained that the previous week had been chaotic, and he experienced complete desperation. He recounted that he intermittently experiences periods of sadness that usually are not caused by an inciting event. He also noted that during these times of depression, his relationships always suffered. The previous week been fighting with his wife over financial and intimacy issues. As a result of the discord, he decided it was best that he leave his home and went to stay with a friend. During this time, James described experiencing emphasized feelings of abandonment and hopelessness. Impulsively, he decided he was going to end his life. He procured some drugs in order to garner the courage to perform the deed. After this, James proceeded to fashion make-shift a noose from ratchet strap he had in the back of his car. He tied the ratchet strap to a pull-up bar in his friend's living room. James's friend was asleep during this time. James proceeded to attempt to hang himself. His friend, however, awoke in the next room. The friend cut James down in time to spare his life.

My attending was able to gracefully extrapolate important details about the incident and gently provided the patient with comfort and reassurance. I was so broken-hearted upon hearing this story from James. I felt so small compared to the suffering the patient was experiencing. I wanted to magically make his problems go away and free him from this burden. All I could do, however, is feel his pain with him. However, from this I took away a few important lessons. First, anyone can be broken, even if they appear composed on the exterior. Second, when I felt powerless in the situation, my attending showed me that even small fragments of encouragement are very powerful. Third, patients are resilient. James initially described his feelings of suffering as insurmountable. By the end of the week, James was looking forward to his future. Lastly, healing from a psychological wound or illness requires work from both the patient and the physician. The patient must be dedicated to trying to heal. The physician must provide the patient with insight, resources, and medication if necessary. I feel that this will make me a better physician as I have learned that any patient can feel helpless and broken no matter what health problem they are facing. I believe that rendering psychological aid is often needed in addition to necessary medical treatments.

A DEVOTED WIFE
EMMA DOYLE (PRE-MATRIC JUNE 2020)

On my first day of preceptorship for the summer pre-matriculation program before beginning medical school in the fall, I am sent to the clinic in a tiny rural town in Western Kentucky. The place is fairly quiet; about half of all visits are now conducted online in light of the recent pandemic, so staff have little need to emerge from their offices. I am meant to shadow a family physician Dr. C, who I have heard is fun and approachable. I enter the doctor's office, which is adorned with photos of her family, antique medicine bottles, and Wonder Woman figurines. Dr. C welcomes me graciously, and after introductions, she shows me just a few feet down the hall to meet her first patient of the day, Mrs. M, who has come for a follow-up appointment after injuring her foot by stepping on some broken glass. Additionally, Mrs. M is scheduled to undergo hand surgery in a few weeks to correct a case of carpal tunnel.

I enter the little white exam room and nervously introduce myself to the patient, telling her my purpose for interviewing her. Within moments of meeting Mrs. M, her quiet and gentle disposition is undeniable. She speaks softly and modestly and trusts me with her story almost immediately; with a reassuring smile in her eye she says she doesn't need to review my work after I have finished. I sit down on a stool opposite of the chair Mrs. M has chosen and begin to take dictation.

Mrs. M opts to avoid telling me about her injuries. Instead, Mrs. M tells me about her life with her husband, and it seems that she has a lot to get off her chest, so I decide not to ask her any more about her medical history than she tells me naturally. Mrs. M makes it clear that almost all of her life has revolved around her husband. Mrs. M dropped out of high school at the age of sixteen to marry Mr. M, who was nineteen at the time. Several years later, Mrs. M. decided to go back to school to finish her GED. Then she went to school again to become a certified nursing assistant. Mrs. M. remembers her time as a CNA fondly. They had four children together, fifteen grandchildren, and enjoyed a happy marriage of thirty-three years.

Toward the end of their marriage, Mr. M developed a severe neurological problem. The couple first noticed that something was wrong when Mr. M started having trouble moving the muscles in his face. In the later stages of his illness, Mr. M.'s shoulder muscles lost almost all their function, and he could also no longer move his chin up from his chest. Mr. M. badly needed full-time care. Mrs. M decided to quit her job as a CNA and took on the full responsibility of caring for her husband, including changing his clothes, bathing, and feeding him.

Mrs. M and her husband lived together in the same house for twenty-three years. They would have lived there longer, but the house burned to the ground in a house fire last September. The couple moved to a new apartment almost immediately. Mr. M's condition deteriorated quickly, and he passed away in the new apartment in January of the following year.

Now, Mrs. M lives alone in the apartment where she struggled with and is still trying to cope with her husband's passing. Her niece and her husband lived with Mrs. M in the apartment for a while, but have since moved out to find a house of their own. Mrs. M has no significant hobbies or recreational activities to take her mind off her grief. Instead, after Mr. M's death, Mrs. M. got a job at the local gas station, where she is now an assistant manager. Mrs. M uses her time at work as a kind of therapy to distract herself. I find myself wanting to encourage Mrs. M to find something that she can do just for herself, but I decide that I don't want to make her feel persecuted, and I allow her to speak. When I ask Mrs. M how her relationship is with the rest of her family, her face visibly brightens around her COVID mask. Mrs. M says that she has a wonderful relationship with her children and grandchildren, and that they visit her often to make sure she is doing okay.

Mrs. M says that has been asked to write a paper about her experience with her husband's illness. Mrs. M takes a long, labored sigh and hangs her head slightly. She says she does not know where she would begin. With a hint of a tear in her eye, she says there is no way to express what it feels like to lose a soulmate. When I ask if she could have any wish granted, Mrs. M. shakes her head and says she only wishes she could have her husband with her again, but that she knows that is impossible. Instead, she hopes that she can keep spending time with her children and grandchildren and making them happy.

After a long pause, and perhaps feeling an air of conclusion, Mrs. M asks me if she told me everything I wanted to know. I told her that if she felt like she adequately summed herself up to me that I had everything I needed. Mrs. M confirms that she has, and I thank her for her time, apologizing that I cannot shake her hand. I try to smile around my mask and quietly exit the room.

I cannot help but worry that Mrs. M is not taking enough time for herself. She is obviously sorely grieving for her lost husband, but she might need other ways to heal besides throwing herself into her work. I imagine, maybe in a way attempting to damper my own concern, that Mrs. M's children will try and encourage her to try her hand at baking or invite her to a yoga class. From what Mrs. M told me, her children seem supportive enough to want to help their mother in that way. Whatever it is, I know that Mrs. M will need to learn take care of herself now that her husband is gone, no matter how strange and difficult that must be for her.

A HYPERMOBILE YOUNG BOY WITH JOY
MARIA SHIELDS (PRE-MATRIC JUNE 2020)

Brayden (not his real name) is a 7-year-old who loves to swim; his mom claims he is "half bullfrog". He loves to go fishing with his great grandpa who is his "running buddy" and fishing partner. Brayden cheerfully recalled the huge fish he saw in the deep end of the pond the last time he went fishing. When he isn't scoping out fish in the pond, he often plays with his cousin Lance outside and has gained a cloak of melanin to prove his adventures outdoors. On the outside, Brayden is an ordinary kid with extraordinary joy.

Brayden has been to nearly 1000 doctor's visits during his short 7 years of life. He was diagnosed with Clostridium difficile colitis when he was 6 months old along with ear problems, a hernia, and an undescended testicle. A few years later, he was diagnosed with asthma at the age of 3 and often had croup. At the age of 4, he was diagnosed with epilepsy and has had over 50 seizures. Thankfully, he has been seizure-free for over a year now. He also has gastrointestinal issues and frequently has constipation and problems with his colon. At the discovery of his primary care physician, Brayden was most recently diagnosed with Ehlers-Danlos syndrome - giving him hypermobile joints and appendages. Although he has never broken any bones, he has dislocated nearly every joint in his body. This is his normal - a simple relocation is enough to send him on his merry way. Brayden "thinks it's cool" that his body can move in such miraculous ways, although his mother disagrees. His childlike joy and fascination with his bodily anomalies was both endearing and pure. How can someone so physically ill be so profoundly happy and content with life? As I watched Brayden wriggle on the exam table, I couldn't help but get the impression that he was a perfectly healthy young boy. How could someone so sick manage to smile and maintain such an abundance of energy? Brayden didn't fit the bill of a very ill child - from the outside he seemed no different than any other 7-year-old boy.

Brayden often dreads going to the doctor. While other kids know every miniscule detail about their favorite cartoon, Brayden has memorized the long white corridors and the locations of laboratories of nearly every facility he has visited. He knows when one simple turn in the hallway is indicative of going to the lab where he will receive the horrible "blood shots". This is what Brayden calls blood draws - an activity with which he has become very familiar. My heart ached at the thought of Brayden wide-eyed with fear as he neared the lab. He travels to the local hospital every 3 months for a follow-up on his conditions. Among his team of physicians are four specialists and his primary care doctor who work diligently to treat his assortment of medical diagnoses. These specialists have known Brayden since he was four months old and they have continued to see him every six months since then. I imagined what it would be like to witness a delicate toddler become engulfed with pain at the hands of invisible illness.

His pulmonologist recently performed a bronchoscopy that revealed highly reactive airways. Throughout the procedure, his tiny lungs were constantly collapsing as if they were gasping for air themselves. He was diagnosed with severe highly reactive refractory asthma - a potential explanation for his constant shortness of breath. As he visits the clinic today, he is being tested for alpha-1 antitrypsin deficiency. This protein is produce by the liver and is crucial to fight off infection and irritants in the lungs. Common complications of its deficiency include chronic obstructive pulmonary disease and emphysema - lung transplants are often common practice for those severely affected. This deficiency is a genetic disorder that is inherited in an autosomal dominant pattern. Interestingly, his grandmother mentions that many other family members have "medical oddities" - some born with one kidney and other missing organs. I wondered if Brayden may have other health conditions influenced by his relatives.

His mom says he often aches at night "like a little old person" which causes him to frequently wake up in pain. As he sits in the comfort of his mother rubbing his feet, he is lulled back to sleep. Despite this common awakening, he is normally the first one awake bouncing around like a bundle of energy. His mother and grandmother both say he is such a happy child; he is joyous and has a love of life. She placed him in head start at the age of one, but he spent more time at home than he did there due to his complex medical diagnoses. He is now homeschooled by his mother who is not only his teacher, but one of his biggest advocates. As they sit on the exam table, he looks up with a toothy grin as he entangles his tiny arm into hers, resting his head against her shoulder. My heart melted as I watched him glance into the eyes of his lifelong protector and friend. As he sat wrapped in his mother's arms, I was reminded of my younger cousin who was born with congenital heart complications. I remember witnessing her mother grieve at the thought of undergoing another surgery. I imagined what it must be like for Brayden's mother, who was undergoing an amplified version of the same type of story.

Brayden's medical conditions are still somewhat of a mystery to medical experts who are often baffled by his comorbidities. Such an array of medical conditions is often not seen until late adulthood, if at all. Unlike these adults, Brayden has yet to experience much of his life. His young eyes have seen, his ears have heard, and his skin has felt more needles than most of us will ever experience in a lifetime. Despite this, Brayden has a contagious smile and a radiating joy that captures the attention of his family and medical providers alike. I have great admiration for Brayden and his unwavering strength. My heart both aches at the complexity of his medical conditions and rejoices that he continues receiving diagnoses that can provide some answer and consolation to his mother and family members. Although a diagnosis may not make his suffering any easier, simply having a name for his symptoms may be enough to comfort his loved ones.

A RESILIENT YOUNG WOMAN WITH A PURPOSE
MARIA SHIELDS (PRE-MATRIC JUNE 2020)

Abby (not her real name) is a 20-year-old college student with big dreams and aspirations to be a veterinarian. She is a sister to four biological siblings. Two are currently in foster care and two that live with her biological father. When she is home for the summer, she lives with her foster mother and two adopted sisters who are biological siblings. She first began living with them when she was 12, but has been in "too many foster homes to count". From the age of 1 to 7, she lived in Arkansas followed by Mississippi where she lived until she was 8 years old. From the age of 8-10, she lived with her biological father. At the age of 10, she arrived in Kentucky where she went into the foster care system again. In addition to the stress experienced from frequent relocation, Abby experienced several years of abuse during this time. Abby was sexually abused while she was in a Mississippi foster home. For the two subsequent years she spent with her father, she was physically abused and spent many days without food and proper care. Thankfully, Abby's teachers recognized this and were able to call Child Protective Services. She has run away a total of three times from two different foster homes, once from a past home and twice from her current foster home. She expresses that she never had control over her life. She has always been told what to do and where to go. All Abby wanted was to make it to 18 years old - then, she thought, she could be free.

Abby is currently home from college for summer break. She meets with her therapist on a weekly basis through telehealth where she has begun her recovery from post-traumatic stress disorder. She not only learns methods to cope, but she also learns techniques to more effectively interact with her family. Between these meetings and the couple of online classes she is enrolled in, she tends to stay quite busy. Not to mention her two dogs who have brought profound meaning and purpose to her life. Abby has a history of self-harming and was able to stop after she got her puppy when she was 16 years old. According to Abby, the dog is stubborn and often talks in her own puppy language - a series of whimpers and noises. She specifically wanted to get a puppy, not a full grown dog because she knew it would require more attention and care. The puppy helped her get out of bed in the morning and gave her a reason to be productive.

Abby says that her current foster home no longer feels like a home. Her younger siblings frequently pick on her and try to start drama within the family. She explains that her mother frequently "sides" with her siblings and claims that it is her fault that she feels as though she isn't part of the family. Last night, an argument began when Abby's siblings told their mother that she was talking negatively about her. Her mom also claims that she has placed voice recorders throughout the home and this is how she monitors what Abby says behind closed doors; Abby doesn't know if she believes this or not. Fed up with her siblings, Abby told her sister to leave her alone and to go "slit her wrists". In retrospect, Abby recognizes that she shouldn't have said this. Following the statement, her foster mother told Abby that she should go and cut her wrists instead followed by telling her to "leave and do not come back" otherwise she will call the police. Abby went to her room and grabbed a backpack, her keys, and her two dogs and left - leaving her shoes and belongings behind. In her bare feet, Abby climbed into her car and began driving without a destination.

It wasn't long until Abby had a panic attack amongst her distress and pulled off on an exit into the gravel. She began cutting her forearms before she called her friend who was able to talk her through things a bit. After she got off of the phone, she continued self-harming. Shortly after, her cell phone lost all service and she was unable to make or receive calls. She believed her mother terminated her cell phone plan. Abby remembered that she could still call 911 without cell service. She called 911 and told the operator that she had cut too deep. Police and EMS were shortly dispatched to her location where they transported her to an inpatient psychiatric unit. Amidst the blue and red glowing lights, the police called her mother to come and pick up the dogs. Abby is deeply concerned that her mother may take the dogs to the pound. She just wants to know they are okay.

Abby is also an avid reader of fiction novels and lover of Marvel movies. Some of her favorite characters are Loki, Thor, Black Widow, and Groot & Rocket. She says Loki often has good intentions but is often misunderstood. He has a comical relation with Thor who often tricks him. At the end of the day, he realizes that Thor really does care about him. She likes Black Widow because even though she has a rough past, she works hard to fix the wrongs in her life and equalize good and bad. As for Groot and Rocket, she appreciates their relationship and their ability to work together and understand each other implicitly. Similar to Loki, Abby is often misunderstood. Similar to Thor, her siblings often "trick" her but there are moments when Abby and her sisters get along with one another. Abby has had a tough past and works hard to improve to her life - similar to Black Widow. Groot and Rocket are like Abby and her puppy. They simply get each other. In her favorite characters, I could see Abby and the types of relationships she values with others.

Abby didn't want to die as she sat in the gravel in the shadow of the exit sign. She was tired of fighting - simply tired of being tired. She didn't feel the pain of the pocket knife as it ran across her arms. Sometimes it feels like she's drowning and can't breathe. For now, she is worried about getting through the next couple of months until school starts back in August. Even if she is able to return to her foster home, she believes it may be best for her to leave for her own sake. She doesn't like looking into the future much because she has been let down too much and has frequently lost hope. Abby doesn't mind telling her story anymore. She's told the story to therapists, doctors, and social workers too many times to recall. Despite the many obstacles and challenges Abby has faced throughout her life, Abby's life has a purpose - one that will influence those around her for years to come. Abby is an extremely strong-willed young lady and we all have something to learn from her resilience and strength.

AN ALL-AROUND HAPPY LADY
EMMA DOYLE (PRE-MATRIC JUNE 2020)

About midway through the morning, Dr. C and I saw our first in-person patient of the day, although we had gone through several tele-visits already, and I am more than ready to see a patient in the flesh. Dr. C shows me into a tiny exam room where Mrs. K sits in a chair in the corner. Mrs. K is wearing bright coral pants and a shirt and wears her graying blond hair in a tightly-pulled bun. She has come to see the doctor for a follow-up appointment to check on the healing progress of a wound on her arm that she sustained in a fall. The wound was wrapped with three large bandages that covered almost the entire length of her arm. After Dr. C and Mrs. K had finished exchanging pleasantries, Mrs. K peeled back the bandage closest to her elbow to reveal an uninfected, cleanly healing wound. "Leave it to a nurse to know how to dress a wound!" Dr. C enthusiastically pointed out, as she gestured for me to come closer to get a good look at the normal healing process. I lean in for a closer look and listen closely to Dr. C's lesson. Although the wound seemed to have been fairly deep into Ms. K's arm, shiny, yellowish tissue indicated that new skin was growing, and punctuated red pin-prick spots were signs that new blood vessels were growing back normally. After the exam, Dr. C excused herself from the room to give Mrs. K and me some privacy for a chat.

I notice Mrs. K's kind and generally cheerful demeanor right away. She is absolutely willing to answer any of my questions. I am thankful she is so willing to help me. When I ask about her life at home, she tells me she has been married to her husband for fifty years, a time which Mrs. K describes as a typical, happy marriage. Mrs. K's husband had a stroke about six months ago, and now she stays home to care for him. They had two daughters together who are now 40 and 42. "They're old like me now," Mrs. K jokes, and I genuinely laugh with her. Mrs. K also has four grandchildren. They only live a half block away from Mrs. K, so she gets to visit her grandchildren often.

As Dr. C mentioned in her examination, I find out Mrs. K is a retired nurse. She went back to school to become a nurse at age 31 after her children were old enough to take care of themselves. Mrs. K first worked as a nurse in obstetrics. I asked her if she enjoyed working with the smallest of children, to which Mrs. K replied, "holding babies is fine, but I don't want to deliver them!" Mrs. K also worked 3rd shift in the intensive care unit. The work was hard in the ICU. Mrs. K tells me she would have to wake her irritable patients up late at night to have them take their medicine. On top of that, Mrs. K often had to tend to fifteen or sixteen other patients each shift, which sometimes made keeping up with her schedule difficult. I momentarily remember my almost debilitating dependence on nightly sleep, and I cannot imagine doing Mrs. K's work. Mrs. K tells me she stopped working as a nurse when her health began to deteriorate.

For the past several years, Mrs. K has developed bronchitis and pneumonia every winter, which has given her considerable fatigue in that part of the year. However, she has not had this problem for the past two years, so she is hopeful that that part of her life is behind her. Mrs. K also underwent a quadruple coronary bypass surgery when she was fifty years old when her doctor discovered that her coronary artery was blocked. I have heard of triple bypass surgeries being performed before, but never quadruple bypass, and I am amazed that Mrs. K seems to have recovered fully from such an intensive procedure. She has had much less trouble with her heart since the surgery. Mrs. K also has trouble with her blood count being too low. She sees the hematologist regularly to check her blood count and takes iron supplements. At one point, Mrs. K's RBCs fell to dangerously low levels, which made her feel seriously ill. She was hospitalized at that point, but soon recovered. To my amazement, Mrs. K tells me she is glad that she had that scare, because at least she knows now what her limits are and when she should seek care.

Mrs. K tells me with a chuckle that she is "definitely not a Type A personality." She loves to lounge in her home and, if given the choice, would sleep until noon every day. When she gets time to herself, she likes to read and watch television. Right now she is watching *Blindspot* and is thoroughly disappointed that the series is not being renewed for a sixth season. She also loves *The Handmaid's Tale* and looks forward to the time when new episodes will be released.

When I ask Mrs. K what she would like her future to look like, she tells me she would have everything be the same as it is now. I am slightly shaken by this unusual response, but I believe her. Mrs. K gives every indication of being a genuinely content person that, despite all her previous illnesses, has led a full life. I tell Mrs. K that her answer is awesome, and I tell her that whatever she is doing, she is doing it right.

Once I make my way back to Dr. C's office, we talk a little more about Mrs. K. I find out that Dr. C and Mrs. K once worked together in the same practice where they became quite familiar with one another. Dr. C describes Mrs. K as a "go-getter" and a "durn good nurse." Although Mrs. K takes full advantage of her leisure time, it seems that she is also a very hard worker on top of her cheerful disposition. I am glad to have met Mrs. K even for a short while, if only to know that some people can remain generally happy in the face of adversity.

BEGGING FOR ATTENTION LEADS TO THE ER JONATHAN SMITH (PRE-MATRIC JUNE 2021)

Miss J is an 18 year old patient admitted to the in-patient psychiatry ward. Born and raised in Western KY, Miss J is one of 7 children born to a schizophrenic mother and a come and go father. She found strength as an older sister to her brothers and sisters, often taking a mother like role in their life. She recognized her mother was overwhelmed and exhausted and knew nothing else other than to do all she could to help around the house. She loved school, graduating from high school in 2020 with plans to go to college. Unfortunately, COVID affected her family as it did people across the country. She felt the need to begin working immediately and forego school so she could help her mother financially. The anxiety and stress of trying to provide for family took its toll, but she persevered and continued to put others first. She met her boyfriend about a year ago and he also works at the same grocery store. She moved in with him last fall to take a financial load off her struggling mother. Trying to provide for brothers and sisters while living on her own was more difficult than she ever imagined. Soon financial stress only increased and arguments with her boyfriend followed. This only brought out skeletons from her past that she was trying to keep concealed. Miss J's mother is a schizophrenic, her father was abusive and left early, and her mother had men around the house that neglected her and the children. Miss J's mother coped with her own struggles with repeated suicide attempts that J witnessed. From a way too early age, she saw her mother attempt to leave everything in order to cope with the struggles this life brought.

Miss J was strong, and she knew it, but the argument last Sunday seemed like more than she could handle. As the argument progressed, she found herself in the kitchen, the eight-inch knife seemed to have stared right back at her. Attempting to gain the attention of her boyfriend, she picked the knife up and went to fake cut her neck. Unintentionally, she got too close and cut a five inch gash in the left side of her neck just missing her carotid artery, barely escaping death. Quickly reality set in, her boyfriend rushed her to the ER and her bleeding was controlled and her laceration was sutured up. A psych evaluation led her to be admitted to the unit that night. Immediately after the knife cut her neck, her eyes were opened to how quickly death could have passed over her and she could have left it all, just like she watched her mother attempt to do so many times. She does not want to be remembered this way and she knows she has so much to look forward to and so many lives to change. Miss J wants to be a therapist, she wants kids of her own, she wants to live a day where she has no financial concerns.

This experience will allow her to connect and talk with those who are going through the most difficult of times, she is able to say the powerful phrase, "I understand you," because she does. Miss J has a heart for the ones searching for their way, indicated by her pet, a recently rescued turtle she found on the road. Miss J loves to read, to paint, and be outside and enjoy nature. She is going to enjoy that much more now with a new lease on life. This is indicated by her voice, her joy that fills the room, and the wisdom that doubles her age. She gained this the hard way, but she has it and wants to share and give it to others. Her story changed my view on mental illness in a remarkable way. We are so quick to judge others based on a snapshot of their life and neglect to view the whole frame. I want to get to know others. I want to get to know patients because everyone is on their own path to happiness and sometimes, they just need help to get back on that path. I only hope to approach others with as much grace as Miss J does. If I ever run into her in the future, I know that she will be everything she ever hoped and dreamed to be.

EXPIRED TOMATO JUICE
HANNAH MARSHALL (CRS JULY 2020)

James presents to Dr. D's office for a post-hospital follow up appointment. I sat to talk with him, but he focused mainly on his interesting condition that put him in the hospital to begin with. James states that a couple months ago he drank expired tomato juice. When I asked how old it was, he joked and said he couldn't tell me because of how embarrassingly old it was. He then states that he got food poisoning from the expired tomato juice and had a few days of bouts of diarrhea and vomiting. After a week and a half, he began to present with a fever and cough and came to the office. Dr. D sent him for more testing, and he found out he had aspiration pneumonia from vomiting over the past couple of weeks.

James was unclear as to how his symptoms progressed, but from our conversation it was clear that his symptoms progressed rapidly. He ended up feeling worse and after calling Dr. D he went to the ER and was admitted to the ICU for almost two weeks with worsening symptoms. James stated that he had never felt worse in his life. After almost two weeks James was discharged from the ICU. Over a week later James stated that he began having diarrhea again and noticed small amounts of blood in his stool. Throughout the day he began noticing copious amounts of bright red blood in his stool and presented to the emergency room again.

They admitted James again and performed a colonoscopy and stool tests and realized he had Cdiff from the antibiotics he was on for his pneumonia. James became severely dehydrated and stated that he was sicker from the Cdiff than he ever was from the pneumonia.

James finally seems to be on the road towards recovery and states that he feels overall well. Despite all that he's been through he states that he is excited to get back to his normal life, free of tomato juice…of course. He states how thankful he is for his wife and family for being with him and boasts that I probably have never heard a story quite as crazy as his.

James's story is one of the most unique stories I may have ever heard. I feel as though it is important to hear stories such as James to understand how to piece things together in complex cases. Although James's story seems like a wild chain of events, stories like James can happen and it helps to understand the complications and probable outcomes of certain illnesses. James's case was extremely interesting to me, and although we didn't spend much time talking about his life or kids or career, I learned a lot about James's perseverance, values, and character in our short conversation.

BIG MIKE AND THE GARBAGE TRUCK
CAITLAN JONES (CRS JULY 2020)

Big Mike was not the least bit what I expected and was the furthest thing from big. In this small town in the western part of Kentucky, everyone knows everyone. This mentality was evident in their community clinic where a middle-aged male patient was simply introduced as Big Mike. Mike was a petite man who works for the city and spends most of his time outdoors. From working with the sanitation department to doing landscaping, his potential roles while working are endless. What brought him in to the office was knee pain that just would not go away. Doing a lot of physical labor, he was not quite able to pinpoint its direct cause. However, he did recall a work accident he suffered a few years ago. While riding on the back of a large garbage truck, the driver was not paying attention and backed up where he shouldn't have. Not only did he hit a minivan, but he pinned Mike in the middle as well. Mike didn't mention what injuries he obtained from the incident, but it was evident how much a life changing experience it was and that he was concerned that this knee pain was related. Mike was a man of very few words and his retelling of that story was the bulk of our conversation. When asked what he wished all doctors did or knew, he couldn't formulate an answer. Likewise, when asked to tell of time when he had a bad encounter with a physician, he also said he couldn't. He said he had never had a bad experience, and that he had a really good doctor. Assuming he was referring to his primary care physician, he expressed how much he liked him and that he had no complaints on the care he had been receiving. Mike was also born and raised in this town and has one son. His son is in his 20s and lives in a nearby town with his mother. The most interesting comment he made during our time speaking was made just before I left the room to get his physician- he didn't have insurance. Without being asked anything about payment or work benefits he threw that short, powerful sentence out as I was reaching for the doorknob- we talked further. He said his work did not provide insurance and that private plans were just too expensive. Mike was there to see a Primary Care Physician who was more than likely going to refer him to see an orthopedic specialist for treatment. A much more expensive visit. He mentioned nothing though of his concerns of affording injections or other treatment, and quickly dropped the insurance conversation. I can't help but wondering though if fear of payment was his real reason for bringing up that tad bit of information in the first place.

At first it was really hard to talk to Mike. He wasn't difficult by any means, just on the shier side. But once I could get him talking about his job, he opened up a bit more. He didn't really like his job, I assume because of the pay and how physically demanding it was. I didn't know what to say when he said he didn't have insurance. The clinic is a community health center with a sliding pay scale and I am sure I had shadowed with many patients who had similar financial situations. But this was the first time I was forced to pay attention to it. I am unsure of why he chose that clinic, but I can't help but think that part of it was because that's the only place he can afford. Every town has hard working men and women that put in 40+ hours a week that don't qualify for Medicaid but also don't have employer based insurance. They need healthcare too.

GAMMA
MATTHEW COLLARD (PRE-MATRIC 2022)

GR is diagnosed with schizophrenia that is reportedly well-managed. She states she does not have cases of paranoia. She was taken to care that resulted in admission to this in-patient psychiatry unit originally by her parole officer. She chose not to disclose any further information about her parole officer or any prior issues with the law. She does not remember the details of coming to the hospital, but she knows that she needs better management of her asthma. She is very adamant on keeping up with the treatment of her asthma and feels that the staff has not helped her with that management.

GR finished high school and did not attend college. She does not remember anything before adulthood, except for "small flashes" of memories from her childhood. She worked for a company that reportedly made clown shoes, toys, and plates and dishes for the hospital in the area. She has not worked in several years. She remembers most of her marriages being "rocky" with "ups-and downs" that eventually led to a divorce. GR states that she enjoyed lots of things when she was younger, including driving around to clear her mind, and still finds the most joy out of spending time with her granddaughter who calls her "Gamma." She also finds enjoyment in making jewelry in her spare time.

GR's life took a turn when her mother died several years ago. She did not want to discuss details, but she says that most of her family cast her out, except for her daughter. She said that some of her sisters used to kick her out of her own house to throw parties without her.

GR's future goals and plans revolve around her daughter and granddaughter. She is very interested in moving to live close to her granddaughter so she can see her every day. It was a pleasure to talk with GR, and I believe this encounter was very meaningful and enlightening. I found that GR has trouble remembering or bringing up topics relating to past trauma. I can tell she is a very family-oriented person, and that the actions and attitudes of her family members play a large role in her mood and well-being. I believe she has a sense that the rest of her family will never allow her back into their lives, or she may never want to be a part of their lives again. She is solely focused on being with her granddaughter, which I believe in part is due to her innocence. Her granddaughter is very young and has no ability to hurt or disappoint her grandmother. I believe past trauma has scarred GR's view of her family and people in general, but I am glad she still holds on to her dear granddaughter and has not lost all hope. She does not seem to find enjoyment in much anymore, apart from the small family she has left.

A GRANDMOTHER WITH BIG PLANS
KENNEDY BREEDING (PRE-MATRIC JUNE 2020)

Mrs. D is a middle aged widow with a kind smile and welcoming aura. She is visiting the clinic due to a pain in her side. She finds this frustrating because she has already had her gallbladder removed and experienced shingles. She says it doesn't feel like the same shingles pain. However, she had no worries coming to see the clinic's doctor whom she called a "blessing" after he took care of her late husband.

Mrs. D's pain has been so severe that she has had to take time off from her work at Walmart. This extended break has resulted in her demotion. However, Mrs. D stays optimistic, saying she doesn't mind spending more time at home because she enjoys seeing her two grandchildren, ages 13 and 18. She then explains how her grandchildren come over when her daughter and son in law go their jobs, also at Walmart.

Also at home is Mrs. D's older sister, who previously lived in an RV with Mrs. D's father. Mrs. D's face lights up as she talks about the RV in which her mother and father used to reside in a "beautiful New Mexico town". However, after her mother died, her sister and father took the RV to

Virginia and stayed with family until the passing of Mrs. D's husband. They then brought the RV to a nearby small town, providing Mrs. D with support and allowing her sister to move in with her and the father to have the RV to himself.

Mrs. speaks fondly of her time with her husband. "We would have been married 41 years this year", she recalls with a smile. Though her husband passed away from cancer 6 years ago, she has kept his dog, a black shih Tzu. He was given to Mr. and Mrs. D when her husband fell ill and their previous dog died. The bond between Mr. D and this dog was evident as Mrs. D recounts the days and nights he spent at the foot of her husband's bed as his health deteriorated. Now she watches after the dog and the two share what she describes as a "love hate relationship." This is due to the dog's need for the constant attention that was previously provided by her husband.

When asked about her ideal future, Mrs. D sees herself in the RV. She perks up as she explains her plans to fix it up once she is retired- a day that was once one year and four months away but she is now unsure of now due to her demotion. She wants to live in it with her dad. Driving it to Virginia to see his family, she hopes to free up time for her sister who rarely gets to see her kids. Mrs. D also wants to cheer on her granddaughter as she pursues her dream of becoming a veterinarian.

Mrs. D is a family oriented grandmother, with a huge heart and a passion for adventure.

RAISED LIKE A WEED
TALIA WOODRUFF (CRS JULY 2022)

A Western Kentucky native and daughter of a WWII veteran. The growing conditions not conducive for warmth and affection. The third child and protector of the eldest sibling who is handicapped. The war was not kind to her father, and he reciprocated those hardships to her and her sister. She did not allow her father to brutalize her sister and often took double the pain. Rape was an unwanted commodity as her father and cousins asserted dominance on her. The social order in southern rural life was the topic of her PhD degree and most of her life where women were

2nd class to men. After a long career and a principal who mimicked her father too closely, she decided to retire. Teaching had been her life and reason to live. Once that dream had ended, she decided to start writing books for children and a book called "Surviving Love in Rural South". Her dreams nowadays are just that to her. She would like to go back to school since being a student is all she knows and lived in a college town. Once she also went to Russia on a mission trip that went badly but this feisty and spunky woman's identity is strongly rooted in her sister. She often calls her sister, and they talk quite a bit. She loves her sister dearly and believes that she is in this world for her sister. Her story is not her diagnosis but rather her upbringing and who she is as a person.

REGRET
LINDSAY TUCKER (PRE-MATRIC JUNE 2023)

Seeing her soft spoken kindness among the morning's chaos, it was no surprise that this woman was a mother of three young children. I quickly learned that being a good mom was the most important thing to her, because it was something that she never had. Growing up, she experienced emotional and physical abuse from her mother who was diagnosed with bipolar 1 disorder. During her childhood, she saw her mom attempt to take her own life three times and saw the consequences of a marriage she described as "toxic." Yet to her, this wasn't the hardest thing she's experienced. Surrendering her first born for adoption at the young age of eighteen was the most difficult thing she's been through. Though she admits her regret today, she cherishes the memories she will make with her five year old daughter and three year old son, who are the lights of her life. Balancing being a single mom as well as a caregiver to her own mother has proven to be a challenging task that she is working daily to be better equipped for both mentally and emotionally. During her time in the hospital, she has had the opportunity to reflect on the past and learn new coping skills for a better future for herself and her kids.

Completing the interview with a patient on an inpatient Psych unit was emotionally difficult but also very eye-opening. I was so appreciative that they were willing to be so vulnerable with me and share their hardest moments. It was the first time I had spoken with someone who had experienced things like child abuse and domestic violence first hand and those topics can be difficult to approach. The interview was a good learning experience for me in that I was able to practice empathy and really think about the perspective of the patient I interviewed. It helped me understand what they were going through and why they were having some of the mental struggles that led them to this.

HELPING OTHERS
MADISON PAYNE (CRS JULY 2023)

At every new event in his life, it was always met with an unfortunate ending. As I sat with my patient, I could not believe the tatters in the life that unfolded right in front of me.

His family was broken. His father left just before he was born, leaving his mother to raise him and three older siblings alone. His family was able to move from project housing when his mother remarried. This step-up would only bring more troubles as this new "father figure" was abusive. School would also be another burden he did not want to bear as he remained truant until high school when another family took him in.

High school was a turning point where he kept up his grades, worked hanging steel, and managed a girlfriend. He smiled as he talked about racing BMX bikes to release everything that he had already been through. After high school, he moved to Las Vegas where he would continue hanging steel. He later became a truck driver and at 27 would meet a woman he would marry later that year.

"Well, that was good!" I said.

"No, it was not", he replied.

His wife cheated on him multiple times. In his words she was a narcissist, and he only stayed with her because of their children. When he would be on the road, he would have constant worry for the well-being of his children. After 18 years he was finally able to separate from her and during that time she turned his children away from him. This is when the drinking began.

"You have to be sober to be considered an alcoholic, I was just a drunk because I was never sober".

Drinking eventually led to a depression where he had a suicide attempt and prayed for a Heaven on the other side. He went into a recovery center, but it led to another attempt. He was able to work his way through a Christian recovery program and it led to 2 years of sobriety.

It was in the visit of an old friend that led him back to today. When he confessed to his Primary Care Physician, he was urged to get help before it got worse. Prior to these events, he was excited to apply for a new position as a counselor to help others who were like him. We discussed how it was incredibly rewarding helping others can be.

I could not believe how he still had such a hopeful outlook on what remained ahead after everything he had been through. All in all, I hope he is successful in recovery and is able to fulfil his wish of helping others.

DON'T FROWN
JESSICA LEWIS (CRS JULY 2023)

Alma (not patient's real name) has been in and out of doctor's offices since she was 12 when it was observed that her pituitary gland was "not in the right place". They discovered that her health issues were due to a tumor pressing on her pituitary gland, which affects all her hormones (some of which have no medication to regulate). The tumor is so embedded in her brain that an operation was determined to be too dangerous. So, for almost all her life she has endured endless amounts of different medications but only minimal improvement in her condition. She battles with hypothyroid symptoms one week and hyperthyroid symptoms the next week. Even though that would drive most people mad, she chooses to look on the bright side because "It could always be worse".

Her childhood was no walk in the park. She is the youngest of nine kids, and the only one with those health issues. Even though she has many siblings, her parents tried to provide as much attention to her health and improving it as possible. A specific memory she has of her mother was when they were on the way to Alma's appointment, and they had to take the bus. Due to her medication inducing a yellow skin change, people were giving her weird looks. Her mother comforted her by explaining they don't understand that she takes medicine that turns her yellow and that it would be okay.

Her condition caused her to struggle in school. She described herself as "erratic and unfocused". She was great at spelling and math, but when it came to other complex subjects, she could not focus long enough to understand it. She knew she would not prosper in the distracting environment of high school, so she got her GED and then completed some college. Instead of feeling sorry for herself because she could not play sports or pursue certain careers, she likes to look on the sunny side of things and treat every day she is alive as a blessing.

She currently works as a Sunday school teacher and prioritizes her relationship with God as the most important. In addition to that job, she tries to go to the church once a week to mop and vacuum the floors. She is not required to do that and does not get paid for it. Doing those chores is a way for her to go above and beyond to support her church and keep it flourishing. When she's not at church, she likes to swim and go see movies with her friends. She also mentioned if given the opportunity to travel anywhere she would go to Italy to admire the exceptional art.

A support system for somebody with a chronic illness is of the upmost importance. Her support system now consists of her stepson, her friends, and God. A significant piece of that support was her husband. They met at a training she was required to do as a new hire at a sales company. She said it was love at first sight. For six years, they were on the road working for that company, but in 1999 they decided to move to Kentucky to care for his unwell mother. They were married for 15 years. They lived there for seven years until he was tragically killed while away on a job. He was in Mississippi after Hurricane Katrina to help with cleanup (as was part of his job) and he was murdered while he was there, and nobody has been convicted. She described him as incredibly kind and selfless. He was killed at 36 years old. She mentioned how July is always a hard month for her and her stepson, especially since this year will be 17 years without him. After he passed, she stayed in Kentucky to raise his son (her stepson), who was 16. He lives an hour away, but they call each other regularly.

Since she has been through so much, I asked her what her best future would look like. She jokingly replied with "getting good sleep and feeling good every day." She then added that if her future is the way it's right now then that would be okay too. She says she's incredibly blessed. She stated that since it takes more muscles to frown than smile, we shouldn't even be frowning. She has an extremely positive outlook on life and does not let anything hurt that.

Throughout her life she has seen an endless number of doctors. When I asked her if she had any advice for someone like me who will end up treating patients one day, she said "listen to your patients. No matter what the bloodwork shows they know how they feel." I will be sure to take that with me when I begin practicing.

This was such a one-of-a-kind experience. Doctors are known to make their visits as quick as possible before moving onto the next one. None of them would have had the time to sit down with her like I did and listen to her life story. I am very grateful I had the opportunity to do this and to talk with such an inspiring woman. I know she will continue to make a positive impact on many more people's lives.

CHAPTER 4
Covid

TV DINNER-WELL DONE
RUSSELL FARMER MD

Good afternoon and thank you for allowing me to serve as your speaker for this Convocation. I am truly humbled to stand here surrounded by so many who were once my students, who I am honored to now call my friends. You have NO IDEA what this honor means to me. If I become emotional or animated during these remarks, please forgive me. Normally, commencement speeches are made by famous people or people who have a large amount of money. They often contain advice, the quality of which can be dubious. Sadly, I am not famous - or rich. And I don't have any new advice this class hasn't heard.

Students, you all have let me and the faculty and staff of the University of Louisville School of Medicine into your lives, and we are so much the better for it. You have worked so hard to reach this moment. I cannot begin to give all of you everything you deserve based on that hard work. So instead, I want to offer my congratulations. And, as a final token of my admiration and appreciation, let me attempt to speak to something that is the absolutely enormous elephant in the room.

You guys have had a hell of a past four years. You don't need me to remind you of all that has happened since you started medical school. What you have achieved represents something exceptional. You undertook the hardest task in all of academia while the world around you burned, and you succeeded. I would like to help your family, friends, and assorted supporters begin to understand what you've been through. Perhaps in doing so, I can encourage each of you to walk a little taller as you come to the stage to receive your hood.

When I sat in my first day of classes in the University of Texas at Houston Medical School, now the McGovern school of medicine, it was a hot, muggy August morning. Each of us showed up to our first day covered in tropical sweat, but eager to learn. Our Dean, Dr. Schultz walked into the classroom in front of all 180 of us. He pushed in front of him a cart full of papers. This was no small feat, as Dr. Schultz was all of 5 feet 0 inches tall and at the time weighed maybe 100 pounds soaking wet. He was roughly 90,000 years old. The term "yoda"-esque comes to mind.

Dr. Schultz was respected by all of us, and it was because of that respect I remember everything he said that first morning with near perfect clarity. You see, Dean Schultz was the paragon of a physician scientist – he had discovered the critical mechanism in the intestine that allowed for the absorption of water as molecules crossed the barrier of the gut. In one swift stroke of combined discovery and genius, he had created the foundation for oral rehydration solution that would one day be marketed to hopeful athletes everywhere as Gatorade. He had also created a cheap, easily producible medication that would save the lives of millions of people afflicted with Cholera. He was quick with a smile, quicker with discipline, and he expected the world from us. We loved him deeply.

The cart that Dean Schultz had in front of him was stacked with papers so high that when behind it, you couldn't see his wizened face. Instead, the Dean of My Medical School was transmogrified into a wisp of grey hair behind so many staples and pages with Xerox black #3 toner ink. Knowing his business, he waited for the laughter to die down. Then, the wisp of hair with old man attached, stepped from behind the papers, floated over to the nearby podium, pulling down the microphone:

"Ladies and Gentlemen" – he paused, and gestured carefully to the large stack of papers next to him for dramatic effect: "The average human being uses around 5,000 to 6,000 words in everyday language. A master of English at his most eloquent uses 8,000, to 9,000 words to create the music that would make angels cry to hear it. Over the course of the next bit, you must learn around 15,000 new words. Most of these words no one here has ever heard before. This morning we will teach you a few hundred words. This afternoon we will teach you a few hundred more. This stack of papers represents what you must learn."

All of us immediately looked at Dean Schultz' cart and papers, shocked at the volume of knowledge we would have to consume and remember in the next four years. There were several audible gasps and one quiet "Oh no!" There was no way we could learn all of that in four years and be functioning individuals. Our brains would fall out of our ears. I turned to the young man sitting next to me, whom I barely knew but would ultimately become one of my groomsmen, "Carter, he can't be serious…" Then the worst happened - Dean Schultz continued.

"This will be a good deal of work for your first semester" and hearing their queue perfectly, the members of the Student Affairs team brought carts upon carts of papers into the lecture hall and parked them next to each other. "This is what I have for you to follow the first semester, ladies and gentlemen." Noticing what I would later learn is my own vagal response, I blacked out immediately.

Upon coming back to consciousness, I learned that three of my classmates had stood up at the end of the presentation and walked out the front door of the medical school never to return. I am NOT making that up. Three people just got up and left. The remaining students then spent the next four years learning all of Dr. Schultz' words. My study partners became my best friends as we learned more words and terms, acronyms, and esoterica than I could have imagined. I have spent the intervening time forgetting many of them, though many remain. The ones that stuck did so because of the wonderful people that taught me how to be a doctor.

My biochemistry professor, who started as Dr. Stroebel, but eventually became "Henry" took me and my friends to live and work for a month in China during my M4 year. He taught me grace, humility, and honesty in the face of my burgeoning confidence. He taught me how to give a proper toast and to use my words well. Alberto Puig who taught me internal medicine on wards – a man of Catalonia so crushingly handsome and blindingly intelligent that he immediately became the center of attention everywhere he went. Nachum Daffney, the Israeli immigrant neuroscientist who led our little group into a new frontier of medical learning called "PBL - problem based learning". These weren't "teachers" in the classic sense. These people became our Sherpas on Everest.

I learned my best medical words from my good friend, mentor, and trusted family confidant Dr. Red Duke. Dr. Duke was somewhat of a legend in Texas, though I doubt many here have heard of him. Equal parts Baptist Minister, Trauma Director, retired tank commander, and philosopher Dr. Duke was who I thought I wanted to be when I grew up. He was the doctor the local news turned to with questions. He brought Life Flight from Vietnam to the civilian world creating the first ever helicopter ambulance for non-combatants. He never let complications get him down. He knew every single person in our hospital by name whether they were the CEO or someone equally as important but with fewer titles and less income. He also had every single one of them on speed-dial. He had the perfect quip for every occasion. He was as if someone had plucked Mark Twain out of time and made him into a trauma surgeon.

Parents, spouses, friends, siblings, and other non-medical folks, let me now address you so you can understand the full gravity of what I am describing. Please imagine with me for a few minutes. Imagine yourself alone. Not a little bit, you're utterly alone. You're in an apartment. You have been told there is a new virus on the loose. You know about viruses; you are learning lots of new virus words. Your new words tell you how dangerous a virus can be. You know enough to be scared in ways that make you very, very frightened; your friends from high school and college don't really understand your fear or why you won't come to a party this weekend. Unlike your neighbors, you know that if you gave everyone you have ever met one metric ton of antibiotics that it wouldn't do any amount of good.

You are learning through your medical words that this virus is going to change everything we know and do. You know before the rest of your friends and family that this disease is going to kill millions of people. And maybe worst of all, you know there is not a damn thing you can do to help. You get to sit there with a screen, not much bigger than a frozen TV dinner while the world you swore in this very room to protect, even at risk to your own life, is burning. You get to sit there in that apartment alone, with that tv dinner screen and worry. And ache. And fear. And through all of that you have to learn Dr. Schultz' words.

Every day another cart comes into the metaphorical lecture hall that is your tiny apartment. You get to learn those words through your tv dinner screen. There are 206 bone words in the human body. There are 600 muscle words in the human body. There are 79 vital organ words in the human body. Except now your cart is a series of electronic files. You go to open the files to see what today's crop has brought. Only there are so many, many new words that your brand-new computer seems to develop some form of computational biliary colic every time you try to open the newest set of things to learn. If this machine sputters, how can YOU be successful? Well, you're not alone…

Every new cartful of words comes with a face. In normal times, this face on your TV dinner would have been your friend. This face, and ones like it, would have taken you to China. These faces would have guided you through to maturity in middle of academic onslaught. They would have taught you the mysteries of life, the universe, and everything at the bedside of the sick and dying. Instead, the face on your tv dinner has been reduced to just that. A face, on a tv dinner. In your apartment. A face saying all of Dr. Shultz's 15,000 words at you.

The words on your screen teach you to worry more. The faces begin to talk about the most important exam of your life which will, unfairly, determine how you can help the burning world outside. You wonder if the world will still be there by the time your turn to help comes. New faces come, sometimes the same face again. And always the face telling you that it wants to help you and be there for you, but it can't because of all the awful words you are learning about. Teaching you the words and world of medicine has been the thing that these people live for. But instead, these would-be friends, mentors, and guides are reduced to faces, saying Dr Shultz' words at you.

You learn new organ words and how each of these organs has an origin in the embryonic cells that develop into what we are. You learn words governing each of these developments and plans for the way the human body works. You learn words for every type of cell and how they look under a microscope, the organelles within them, the proteins governing their function, and the signals all these tissues send to each other; once you know those words, you get to learn a whole new category of words.

The faces begin to teach you that your new words have MORE new words simply made up to describe the first set. You're positive that a sarcomere is actually the name of your favorite dinosaur you learned as a child. The faces tell you every way every single one of your new words can become deleted, blocked, inhibited, up regulated, phosphorylated, de-phosphorylated, re-de-un-ultra-phosphorylated, stimulated, action potentiated, assayed, and on.

And on.

And on.

You learn the words of microscopic bodies. You must know about all of these invisible creatures and how they work. The faces say that knowing about the small body words can keep you from being sick. You must know which little wee beasties cause what disease and in what presentation. You must know how many different diseases can come from the same little beastie in its various forms. Which one does the spleen kill? Why not others? So many tests, all online. Things begin to mush together. So much, nonstop, so, so much.

Now family members, spouses, friends and guests, with that backdrop, imagine that this is every day, for hours uncountable. The tv dinner drones and outside the world burns some more.

You get words that someone with a broken typewriter just made up one afternoon to slap on a chemical with a million side effects. You get to know the words for drugs that other people don't get to know. Magic, secret words that indicate you're a knower of deep knowings! Forget saying "asprin"! Now it's acetyl-salicylic-acid. One face says that if you want to be cool you can say "ASA". Words. More words. Words with so many letters your head hurts to hear new ones from the face on the tv dinner. Words never ending…words enough to make 3 people get up and leave after simply finding out how many words there are…

Time slows to a crawl. Words are everywhere, tiny biting midges in a bog. The burning world begins to cool slightly, only to backdraft again. And again. You wonder if you're dreaming. How many more faces? You start to think that maybe the medical school has hired a rogue etymologist to create these words and they are just messing with you. Your friends are faces. Your classmates are faces. Is this real? How many more faces and words can there be?

Feeling equal parts crazy and alone, it would have been easy to give up. It would have been easy to do what my classmates did – just up and leave. Quitting would have been understandable. After all, you have the perfect out! Deadly virus? Years of isolation? Who on earth could blame you? Take your talents and do something else to make your family proud. It would be so......easy.....But you didn't. You thought of your patients, and your duty. You looked at the burning world outside, and the nurses and doctors dying, and families saying goodbye over iPads, and not enough PPE, and who knows what else.

You saw every one of those things, and you know what you said? Do your parents, friends, and communities know what YOUR words were when faced with those evils? What did you say when millions were dying? You said, "I'll learn your words, all 15,000 of them. I'll learn whatever the hell a Coronavirus is and I. WILL. FIGHT. IT. I am READY. PUT ME IN, COACH." You didn't give up.

You never, ever, ever, ever gave up.

Despite every adversity, you came out from behind the tv dinners and faces, and you brought your words back to bedside where they belong. You fought and clawed your way past COVID, and STEP, and ISOLATION, and RACIAL TRAUMA, and the LOSS OF FAMILY, and innumerable blockades against your will. And through that fight you mastered this massive new vocabulary and made it yours. I know because I have heard your words at the bedside of your patients. Your colleagues have heard those words echo in their ears as you have matured and become the doctors you were ALWAYS meant to be. Your words are power. Your words are those of a generation of warriors. Your words have transcended a cart of papers with floating grey wisps of hair. Your words are the music that makes angels cry just to hear it.

The day will come over the next years or decades when you feel as if you may as if to falter. A beloved patient may die. Your treatment plan will not achieve the desired outcome. The electronic medical record will be itself and you'll have to survive it. I pray in those moments of self-doubt that you can think of the strength you have displayed before all of us that have believed in you. I hope you can lean on remembered strength in those days and be proud of it in the happier moments. The cart with the words will always keep coming, but now you are the master of the cart and its contents. Heck, some of you might make some new words the rest of us will get to learn.

My dear friends and colleagues; when you come to the stage today, please, I beg you stand tall. Stand tall and receive the honor that is due to you. Face your families and friends with as much pride as you can. Then go back and find some more. Generations of students have graduated from the UofL School of Medicine; but there is NONE that has achieved what you have. Stand atop this summit and gaze down at how far you have come. And if you ever need to lay down your packs, I promise that the faculty and staff at the UofL SOM will always be here to serve as Sherpas for your next climb.

It has been among the great honors of my life to serve as your speaker. It has been an even greater honor to see you grow into such strong, intelligent young physicians. I do not exaggerate when I say I love every one of you from the very, very bottom of my heart. I will leave you with one last thought. Many people argue over the most powerful word in English language. Some say "Yes." Or they say "I will" or any number of variations on that theme. However, I might assert that there is no greater word for relieving pain and suffering, for healing, and for hope beyond the word it is now my absolute privilege to call all of you, from this moment forward: "DOCTOR".

STEPPING UP TO THE PLATE
SARAH FISHER, MD

As a newly graduated OB/Gyn resident, I was fortunate to be able to come back to the hospital in my hometown as my first attending job. This is the same hospital where I spent the last two years of medical school. This is the hospital that hosts all of the memories that made me fall in love with obstetrics and gynecology. This is the hospital where I see the nurse who I've known my whole life when I see patients. This is the hospital where I remember making "rounds" with my dad at age five. Returning to practice in Madisonville has been a pleasure, but it certainly has had its difficulties.

I love having known my general surgeons since they were my attendings in medical school. But every time I operate, I wonder if I'm good enough to be in the operating room next to them. I enjoy seeing smiling faces walking in to work and saying hello to the nurses who taught me to put in a Foley catheter, but I hope they don't think I'm too young to take care of their patients. I am proud to be a female physician but I fear that when administrators look at me, they see an outspoken "dumb blonde" female physician. Being a new attending just out of residency is challenging as we overcome imposter syndrome, eventually realizing that all of those years in residency did in fact teach us a thing or two.

Now throw in COVID-19. In my first year out from residency, I had no idea that a worldwide pandemic would turn my own world upside down. In February, my biggest concerns were upcoming oral boards, teaching medical students, and making sure that I didn't kill a patient. Then came March 2020. Suddenly, I worried if I was safe around my patients – or if they were safe around me. Did I carry the virus? Would I infect my patients? My surgery patients didn't understand cancelling their hysterectomies, sobbing on the phone; I can see how their "elective" surgery doesn't seem elective to them. I was not trained how to handle this and "Pandemic 101" was certainly not part of the residency curriculum. The most dramatic change that I experienced was my role as a physician. Not only was I voyaging into the world of telemedicine, but also making big decisions about our Labor and Delivery unit. With my two partners, we decided how we would handle a COVID patient in labor and during delivery, advocated for fit testing for all of our staff, and urged all to wear N95 masks during the second stage of labor and during delivery to protect ourselves. I streamlined a policy for mother and baby bonding after delivery for COVID patients with approval from my partners and our neonatologists. More than once, our labor and delivery nurse manager asked, "Dr. Fisher, what do you think?" I realized that as a rural physician, I was being turned to for advice and guidance on how to handle this unprecedented pandemic. It didn't matter that I was green and had virtually no experience under my belt. I was still viewed as a leader.

While I felt the weight of this pandemic, I have been reminded of the vital role of the rural physician. This is not just from a patient care perspective but also from a process and policy standpoint. We are viewed as the leaders of healthcare in our communities and that responsibility should not be taken lightly. In times when our staff and patients need an advocate, we are responsible for stepping up to the plate and answering the call. Not only do we comb through every CDC guideline and expert opinion to provide the very best care for our patients, we also are involved with developing and modifying policies to keep our staff and patients safe. I thought I needed experience to make a difference; really all I needed was heart. While my rural hospital may not have initially sought a green female doctor to answer their call for a leader, I feel lucky to serve my community in a unique way.

COVID 66: ARE WE TOO OLD FOR THIS?
BILL CRUMP, MD

As I drove in to make weekend rounds at our hospital, I noticed a buzzard circling above. It gave me pause. Well, I thought, at least it's just one buzzard. This whole social distancing thing has shaken me to my core.

As I passed my 65th birthday and watched all the subspecialists around me retire, I really had to stop and think what I would do if I no longer saw patients. And then I realized that at 65 our hospital bylaws said I could stop taking hospital night call. Fewer nighttime awakenings seemed like a good idea after 22 years of 24 /7 call backing up our residents' deliveries. But it slowly dawned on me that if I stopped taking night call and with younger faculty now available, it didn't seem reasonable for me to do daytime deliveries and ask them to do those at night. With that, a part of me that had been so integral stopped as well. I still oversee prenatal care with the residents, but have stopped doing deliveries. Life was less complicated, and I felt more rested and able to give my daytime work my full attention.

And then this confounded virus. Initially the CDC said that high-risk groups were older age and underlying conditions. I heard this three times from the same NIH official in the same day. Then somehow over the next few days their recommendations changed from "and" to "or". Suddenly, those of us with gray hair and perhaps some wisdom to share become at risk by doing what we've done every day for almost 40 years.

As we wait to see if the plague strikes our small regional hospital, disappointment is the reigning theme. I was scheduled to receive a national medical education award for our campus at the meeting in my hometown of Savannah. Family could attend and it seemed like a nice inflection point in my career. On the same weekend I could see my granddaughter play soccer in a tournament that is worthy of her Olympic development team skills. I could visit with the family and walk through the Cathedral, the squares downtown, and all of the places that made me who I am.

Meeting canceled, travel advisory for anyone my age, trip canceled, and disappointment. As we all struggle to decide what parts of medical education should still continue and whether we could possibly have any resident or medical student conferences with 6 feet between each learner, it suddenly dawned on me that I may be at risk in my own hospital.

I provide medical support for our inpatient geriatric behavioral health unit. What should I do the next time I'm called about a patient with fever and a cough? I could do a lot of the evaluation by video, but I'm just old-fashioned enough to need auscultation to help me make decisions. Although I used telemedicine auscultation 25 years ago with NASA, there's no quick way to set it up in our small hospital. And then there's the experience I had this morning. A woman just a few years older than I had been admitted for worsening dementia and some verbal aggression. As I examined her, she ruminated with wild eyes on who would put her in such a place and asked me every few seconds how she could get out.

No verbal reassurance worked, but when I just held her hand and told her how much we cared and how her family had entrusted her to our care, she visibly relaxed. There is no way we could have gotten to that first step of healing by video.

For those of us over 60 but still in good health and thrilled every day to see patients and interact with learners, what do we do? There are no clear guidelines. As I often do, I harken back to my mentor Dr. Gayle Stephens, who was one of the founding fathers of family medicine. Paraphrasing the central tenet of his philosophy: the definition of a family doctor is one who cannot ignore any issue brought to him by his patient.

I am going to find a way to get through this without losing who I am. And buzzards be damned.

EMERGENCY USE
BILL CRUMP, MD

General Washington saw it as a sign of weakness

And bore the scars

It was still experimental and strange it seemed

A simple scratch to protect an army?

Worth a try if hidden from enemy prying eyes

But at Valley Forge a last resort in full view

Masks not even a thought

And quarantine a reverse miasma

Psalm 91 says not to fear

Angels won't allow you to strike your foot upon a stone

But was it an angel of fear who guided Jenner?

The father of our country would say surely not.

During the critical part of the revolutionary war, Washington discovered that many of the British soldiers had been exposed to smallpox as children and therefore were immune. He realized that his forces were being decimated by this infection, as many of the colonists had not had previous exposure. Washington himself had contracted the disease in Barbados 25 years earlier, leaving him with a small scar on his nose. Quarantine was known to be effective, but was very unpopular and simply could not be enforced in tightly packed encampments. The irritation of quarantine was confounded by the prevailing concept at the time that plagues were spread by a cloud of evil termed a miasma. Variolation was established almost 20 years before Edward Jenner's landmark paper showing that inoculation with cowpox could prevent smallpox. The procedure during the time of Valley Forge required taking a small amount of exudate from a smallpox lesion and placing it in a scratch on the soldier's arm. The result was a very mild illness but sometimes quarantine was still suggested. Reports from the time show that Washington believed that if the enemy knew this process was going on with his army, they would know to attack while the Continentals were weakened. So he sent waves of his army away for this to occur, unknown to the enemy. In the truly desperate days of Valley Forge, he changed this policy to include variolation within the encampment.

The risk of this procedure for "emergency use" was that it would cause an outbreak within the encampment. In one of Washington's letters, he said he feared the disease more than the sword of the enemy. He accepted the risk, and the rest of the story, as they say, is truly history.

FEAR ALL AROUND
TRAVIS WHEELER MD, COMMUNITY PRACTICE

Everyone's world has been turned upside down in the wake of COVID-19. As physicians, we have been tasked with navigating an ever-changing situation. As a Family Physician in an ambulatory office, I see and hear the fear expressed by patients who look to my colleagues and me for answers. We as healthcare providers experience a different kind of fear and anxiety knowing that the information we are providing is simply the best information available at a given moment. The "right" answer is constantly changing. I try to offer reassurance to those with mild symptoms, try to protect my elderly or ill patients by keeping them out of the office when possible, and try to manage my own anxiety with the uncertainty of the situation. Never in my career have I second-guessed my medical decision-making as much as in the current pandemic. We are all trying to figure out how to manage the situation safely and effectively. In an effort to try to prevent potential exposure to our patients, the network for which I work, like many others, very rapidly implemented telemedicine visits. Instead of having patients come to the office for acute or chronic concerns, we are now able to provide medical care via telephone or video visit. This technology was deployed rapidly in an effort to maintain access to healthcare for our patients. Technology that typically would be introduced over the course of months was set into action in a mere 72 hours. In my office, I took the role of educating my partners on how to utilize the telemedicine technology and developed an office workflow plan to facilitate smoother implementation of telemedicine visits for our front desk and clinical staff.

We are in uncharted waters. Every day is a new set of fears, anxieties, and uncertainties. We didn't necessarily sign up for this; potentially to put our lives and the lives of those we love on the line to care for others, but we do it. We do it because we are Family Doctors. We didn't sign up to walk into each exam room, clad in surgical masks, countless fears swirling in our mind, asking "am I going to miss the diagnosis of Coronavirus in this patient?" "Am I, as a young, healthy physician, possibly an asymptomatic carrier, indirectly exposing my patients and family?" "How do I decide who should and should not be tested when constantly reminded of the severe shortage of tests?" Further, we are frequently reminded that due to shortage of tests and PPE, we are practicing outside the normal Standard of Care.

In most situations, coming home after a long day at the office offers a sense of reprieve and relaxation. Unfortunately, however, during the current pandemic, coming home has its own stressors. I pull into my garage, immediately remove any clothing which may have been exposed to the environment, go inside, change my clothes, wash my hands, and THEN greet and hug my husband. I constantly worry about the possibility of exposing a family member to coronavirus as a by-product of my career. I worry that my mother who has a chronic respiratory illness will contract coronavirus. Not to mention trying to process the constant barrage of new information from countless work emails, news reports, and social media. It is proving harder and harder every day to find a way to relax, detach momentarily, and unwind.

In light of it all, however, we remain flexible, we adapt to our ever-changing landscape, and we do what is needed to provide the best care possible for our patients and those we love. Because we are Family Doctors.

SUPERFICIAL INTERACTIONS WITH UNSURE ANSWERS
STEVE ROBY MD, COMMUNITY PRACTICE

COVID 19 has been a liminal period of uncertainty and adaptation. It is a virus that has affected everyone and nearly every aspect of society. We've all been stressed with this, trying to figure out how to be and what to do, and frustrated by the many life-altering changes that have been required. It's been tough not seeing our families and friends. It's been tough not having daycares or babysitters to help with our kids. As I write, many areas are beginning to reopen slowly. Yet after over a month of "social distancing" and self-quarantine, we still struggle to judge the best way forward.

I didn't initially realize how big a deal COVID 19 was going to be. I thought it might be like a bad flu season. But it slowly became obvious that the virulence and potential lethality of the illness was too much to abide the status quo. At first, there were plans from the governor to cancel unnecessary procedures. Then recommendations to avoid groupings of over 50. Then advice to avoid groups of more than 10. The guidelines changed daily, yet at times, they seemed out of date. Churches closed. Restaurants closed. In my primary care practice at a small private group, we tried about 1 week of intensive triage at the front door before switching to telemedicine completely.

At first, seeing patients through a computer screen was awkward, although I adjusted. Physical exams and treatment plans were trickier at times, and on average, encounters seemed a little more superficial. The lack of non-verbal cues and physical presence really made a difference. You can't pass a box of Kleenex through the phone to a grieving widow the way one might in the office. I noticed it while trying to manage a conversation on speakerphone with multiple family members, or counsel elderly patients who weren't quite sure what medicines they were on. Some of the dialogue slowed down, and I found myself using short, simple questions as if I were speaking through a translator.

Still, it was nice not to have to worry as much about contracting COVID19 myself. I didn't want the virus, and didn't want to bring it home to my family. The telehealth visits were certainly better than nothing, and most patients were grateful. It was nice to be home with my family a little more, although it was stressful at times too. At times, I'd be conducting a telehealth visit in one room of our house while hearing our 2-year-old have a temper tantrum in the next. He was off his routine too.

I would potentially face the virus again on my turn for hospitalist week. And there was paperwork to be signed (how long does it live on paper?) and groceries to get. My patients asked if it was safe to take ibuprofen and asked about COVID causing blood clots. They wanted to know if it was safe to go to a public park and when would this be over. One woman I saw learned she had COVID right after learning she was pregnant. She didn't feel well and was certainly anxious. I gave each of them the best advice I could. At times, I had to find the answers, other times answers didn't seem to exist. The uncertainty was frustrating, and some of the anxieties of my patients rubbed off on me. But I realized that like Simon of Cyrene, I really was helping people, lightening their burdens just a little, bearing some of the weight for a moment, helping them forward, messy though it may be. Hope prevails.

As of our last meeting, the pregnant woman was doing fine.

HISTORY IS IN THE MAKING
REBECCA RAJ MD, COMMUNITY PRACTICE

As an Internal Medicine resident physician in Milwaukee, Wisconsin, I have felt fearful, uncertain and yet protected as a learner with the reports of the ongoing COVID-19 pandemic. Like a storm blustering its way across the world, I remember reading about the disaster first in China, then Italy and before long in New York, thinking surely Wisconsin will be next. Would the reduced travel and social distancing work? Will we have enough PPE to protect our patients and ourselves when we reach a peak number of cases? At the time of my reflection, our state's Department of Health Services is reporting 12,543 confirmed cases, 6,542 recovered cases, and 453 deaths, equivalent to a 4% mortality and 54% recovery rate. We are also 54 days from the issuance of the governor's stay-at-home order and 4 days from the order being overturned by the Wisconsin Supreme Court. The limits of our healthcare system are being challenged and history is being written right before my eyes. I have been eager to work alongside my colleagues and the words of Esther from the Bible come to mind, "Perhaps you were born for such a time as this."

What we were learning about the virus in early March was rapidly changing which was reflected in our protocols shifting from a daily to sometimes hourly rate. I had the privilege of caring for patients in the emergency room as we began to see a rise in patient cases and what I found was that it is the hard times in life when our strength is tested and our hope in humanity is renewed. What follows are a few interactions that have stood out to me as a testament to the perseverance people exhibit during times of peril.

A single mother of 9 was receiving pantry support from her faith community and was told to get tested before they would continue providing supplies. She risked coming to the hospital and went through the long triaging process before I met her sitting with a mask in the ER bed. Unfortunately we did not have enough testing kits to offer testing to asymptomatic patients. While she was turned away, we did provide an informational packet that would hopefully help her to continue to receive resources. I felt helpless because our job is not just about keeping patients safe and healthy; this pandemic has affected the socioeconomic aspects of every hard working family in America.

As such, it is not only the COVID-19 patients and their families suffering. In the ER bed next door, an older gentleman sat looking pleasant and somewhat confused. After glancing at his vitals and labs, I knew he would be admitted for decompensation of his chronic illnesses. His nurse asked me to talk to his wife in the waiting room since visitors were not allowed beyond the triage station. With tears in her eyes, his spouse shared that they had been married for 46 years and that she has been at his bedside for every hospital admission for the last 20 of them. I reassured her as best as I could but I knew she would still go home fearing for his safety. I was left wishing that I - as a medical caregiver - could do more for this woman beyond the sympathetic smile behind my mask and the bumping of elbows. I do not think I will underestimate the value of a handshake or hug ever again.

Everyone is persevering in different ways during this season including local businesses, hospitals, and whole communities. I'm inspired by my mentors who have been working tirelessly to ensure patient safety and effective communication between departments despite the influx of changing guidelines. Nobody could have predicted the impact of this virus but seeing the community come together gives me hope that we will be stronger when the storm finally passes. I hope that like a phoenix rising from the ashes, healthcare as we know it in the US will be reborn to better serve the very same individuals that came together during this pandemic. As the whole world was brought to its economic knees without the firing of a single bullet, this experience definitely illuminates the deficits in our current healthcare and government systems. We as a nation must come together before history repeats itself.

EFFECTS OF COVID-19 ON PRIMARY CARE
SUMMER SPARKS (CRS JULY 2020)

For many primary care physicians, COVID-19 has affected the quality of the services they can provide in many ways. Many non-essential health care facilities temporarily closed at the beginning of the pandemic, but most primary care offices remained open in order to accommodate their patients who may need to access services, despite government recommendations. This placed emphasis on the importance of primary care and the level of devotion primary care physicians have for their patients and communities. Primary care physicians have remained on the front-line throughout the course of the pandemic and have courageously embraced this formidable responsibility.

Not only did the workload for primary care physicians increase, but it also affected how physicians interact with their patients. It is often important for physicians to build trust and show empathy toward their patients.

Empathy is most frequently displayed though body language, a smile or a handshake but are not permitted currently due to the strict safety precautions that must be followed. Because physicians must wear masks during an office visit, it has also decreased efficient communication between patient and physician. Many patients who have hearing impairment have difficulty understanding important information and instruction provided by their physician because they are unable to read their physician's lips. Overall, social distancing has contributed to a more impersonal method for treating patients.

Many practices, however, did not see patients in person at all and switched entirely to a form of telemedicine. This resulted in some positive and negative consequences. Mainly, telemedicine provided physicians a safe and convenient opportunity to treat many of their routine patients that otherwise would have been unable to come in for a visit during the pandemic. Telemedicine also allowed many patients to have the ability to ask their physicians questions, have their medications adjusted, and discuss new complaints. Many patients with busy schedules seemed to find telemedicine to be actually more convenient than office visits especially for minor complaints and routine check-ups. Physicians, however, are still struggling with technology issues on a daily basis. Often internet connection is poor, and buffering occurs making communication fragmented and difficult to understand. Another issue with telemedicine is that some patients cannot access the necessary devices required in order to complete the televised visit. Some did not have access to routine screening or lab work during this time resulting in poor health outcomes. Representatives from pharmaceutical companies also were unable to provide samples to physicians. This also proved to be detrimental for patients because they were unable to try potentially helpful medications for no cost.

Although these regulations were and still are necessary to reduce the spread of COVID-19, mandatory social distancing has also further isolated elderly populations and increased a sense of fear and hopelessness in immunocompromised patient populations. It has also weighed heavily on physicians because many believe that they are unable to have close relationships with their patients.

I think that it would be extremely difficult for me to feel as though I could not effectively communicate with my patients, that alone would be frustrating and dangerous. I think also that many physicians feel guilty and powerless because they are not able to provide as much emotional support as they could prior to the pandemic. I am interested to see how medicine will continue to progress post-pandemic. In the future, I think that the use of telemedicine will be available to those who wish to conveniently see their physician. However, I think that also physicians will never again take for granted a hug or a handshake. I think that healthcare providers have been reminded through this experience that the reason they work every day is to build bonds with their patients that will result in improved qualities of life.

REMAINING HOPEFUL FOR THE SAKE OF PATIENTS SUMMER SPARKS (CRS JULY 2020)

The 2019-2020 COVID-19 pandemic has posed a number of new challenges for physicians. Physicians not only must balance patients who may be positive for COVID-19 along with all their routine patients. Physicians are also belabored with many regulations that they must follow in order to keep themselves and their patients safe. Many physicians claim that safety regulations such as wearing a mask and social distancing make them feel disconnected to their patients. Nonverbal communication is impeded by masks and physicians and patients have a more difficult time communicating.

Although these new regulations are mandated to keep the population safe, they can have both positive and negative effects on patients. Some patients are put at ease knowing that they are entering a health care facility that follows safety guidelines. These restrictions also help limit the possibility of the health care providers becoming ill with the virus. It appears that patients seem to be compliant with the guidelines. However, the safety regulations may also have detrimental effects on patients. Many patients may feel more isolated from others. Also, many may feel more anxious and the strict protocol may make them feel uneasy.

Because a pandemic is stressful, it has been the cause of many stress-related health concerns that physicians may be presented with. Primarily, patients are simply worried about acquiring the life-threatening virus and the health of their loved ones. Many are also plagued with the fear that they may not be able to support themselves and their dependents if they were to become ill. Because of this worry, patients may exhibit lack of sleep, difficulty concentrating, worsening mental health issues, and/or an increasing in alcohol, tobacco, or drug use. All of these issues are of concern to primary care physicians. Physicians must be prepared to counsel their patients on healthful coping techniques during this difficult time. Some coping techniques may include getting rest, connecting with loved ones, proper nutrition, and exercise. Physicians may also be prepared to grief counsel those of their patients who have lost loved ones due to this pandemic

Physicians are elite problem-solvers. The COVID-19 pandemic, unfortunately, does not currently have a viable solution. This is extremely frustrating to physicians. Although physicians cannot produce a cure or vaccine currently, they must continue to perform their job the best to their ability and remain hopeful for the sake of their patients.

From shadowing many physicians during College Rural Scholars, I got to see first-hand how rural primary care physicians are handling COVID-19. Many are having to see fewer patients due to decreased staff and technical difficulties due to telemedicine. At some facilities in Muhlenberg County, many of the providers are ill with the virus and have had to take a leave of absence. Because of this, some facilities are short-staffed, and the remaining providers have had an increased workload. It is admirable that many providers have stepped up to help their colleagues and patients during this difficult time. Physicians are also doing the best they can to give the best quality of care possible given the circumstances. These providers in the community have stepped up to take on a task that is not easy. This requires a great deal of courage and selflessness.

ARE SPORTS THAT VALUED?
CAITLAN JONES (CRS JULY 2020)

Testing. After social distancing and the wearing of masks, testing seems to be the next most talked thing in regard to the COVID-19 Pandemic. Antigen testing is an interesting phenomenon due to its seemingly lack of availability and efficiency to the masses, and the opposite in the sports realm. To further explore this double standard, let us explore testing at a small community health center in Providence, Kentucky and in the National Basketball Association's "bubble" in Orlando, Fl.

Health First Community Health center resides in a town of just a little over 3000 people. Many locals are employed at large factories and have pre-existing health conditions. However, there is only one testing site in the entire county. This clinic though is trying to address the problem of unavailability by spearheading a mobile testing site in a camper trailer. However once this process began, another issue arose- efficiency. The clinic is in contract with one medical test provider and therefore was required to consult with them first. Although they originally thought timely tests were possible, the testing option they provided was anything but. Currently, the testing service they are able to provide has a ridiculous turnaround time of 14 days. Not knowing if one is positive or negative for two whole weeks serves almost no purpose. Luckily though, the clinic coordinators are in the works of securing another testing service provider that can get results back in 48 hours. The point though, is that it is difficult to provide adequate testing in rural communities. It is expensive and can become a long-complicated process when the business aspect of medicine gets in the way and money isn't in an abundance.

On the flip side, the NBA is testing patients like it's as simple as weighing them. Currently, the association has created a "bubble" in an effort to resume the 2020 season. In order to play in the upcoming games that start back on July 30th, players must remain inside the set barriers and not have any outside contact. If they do, they must quarantine for a 10 day period. While in their designated Disney resort locale, players are not only tested, but tested *nightly*. Once the season is in action, roughly 300 players will get tested 7 days a week. In the professional sports realm, neither availability nor efficiency is an issue. But also, money is not an issue. A multibillion-dollar network like the NBA can afford to get quick accurate results with no issues what so ever. Between the forced social distancing and continuous testing they are hoping to create a safe environment so that a 2020 NBA finals champion can be named.

The overall goal of COVID-19 testing is to better the health of the one being tested and the community as a whole. However, not all individuals and communities are afforded the same opportunities and thus the same health outcomes. This comparison is thought provoking to say the least and begs the question: Do we really value sports that much more than anything else?

I am an avid sports fan and have mixed emotions on the return of major sports like the NBA and the MLB. I am glad to be able to watch sports, but I get aggravated at the amount of tests they are using. Just imagine if the same number of swabs went out to the public and if the NBA used their funds to sponsor widespread mass testing. College campuses can't test returning students periodically, but they test athletes biweekly. Something isn't adding up, and it needs to be addressed.

PATIENT CARE BEHIND THE MASK
CIERRA WOODCOCK (CRS JULY 2020)

The COVID-19 pandemic is single-handedly responsible for making doctor-patient relationships more difficult than they have ever been. Many difficulties in patient care have presented themselves since the rise of the pandemic this year. When everything shut down, doctors were unable to see patients face to face, "elective" procedures were cancelled, labs and imaging were not conducted, and treatments were not received.

Doctors not being able to see patients face to face seemed like an easy fix, with the growing popularity of telemedicine, doctors can simply call their patients via video chat, call in a prescription, and be done. This can all be done without the doctor ever physically touching the patient. Now, this idea sounded great in theory, but in practice both doctors and patients seemed to favor in-person visits more. Many patients said they felt that their quality of care had decreased due to the doctor not being able to physically see or touch them. It does not take a rocket scientist to know that what can be seen in a video is not as reliable as seeing it with your own eyes. Doctors agreed with patients, stating they felt that they were not able to give their best care and were afraid they would miss something on the virtual visit that they would not miss in an office visit. One doctor even said, "The physical exam is one of the most important parts of practicing medicine. Without it, a lot of things can be missed."

Also, as part of not being able to be seen in person, patients were going without things they needed simply because they were considered "elective." One patient had gone without her B12 shot for two months, another had her knee replacement cancelled and rescheduled twice, another was supposed to have bariatric surgery but had to have it pushed back because she was unable to complete her check-ins. People complained that they had increased levels of pain, depression, anxiety, and felt less healthy than they had before all of this had started. Patients hated not being able to see their doctor when they needed to.

Once offices opened back up and patients were able to be seen again, life still did not return to normal. Now, everyone is required to wear a mask, six-foot social distancing has been put in place, and the number of people that can gather at a time has been decreased to a minimal number. Patients and doctors alike dislike wearing the masks because they feel it takes away the personal component of the doctor patient relationship. It is impossible to see facial expressions and words are often miscommunicated. Patients often thought the doctor was upset with them simply because they were talking louder so they could easily be heard. The best thing that describes the effect of the masks on doctor-patient relationships was from a doctor saying, "They can't even see my smile, so they know I care and I'm happy to see them."

Overall, COVID has had an extremely large negative impact on doctors and patients alike. Both are ready for all of this to come to an end so that healthcare can return to the way it was before. Most patients and doctors think that it will only come to an end when a vaccine is developed, but that seems to be years away. Hopefully, it will be over soon enough so healthcare can do what it does best—improve the quality of patients' lives.

At first, I thought that all of this was only hard on the patients. However, when I spoke to the doctors, it seemed to be just as hard on them. Well, at least for the ones that truly care about their job and patients. Seeing the way these doctors felt and the way they advocate for their patients was astounding. As a future physician, it motivated me to be the doctor that does everything they can to alleviate patients' suffering, whether it be physically or mentally. Doctors that truly care about their job, care about their patients and want to provide the best quality of care for them.

NURSE'S PERSPECTIVE ON COVID-19 CIERRA WOODCOCK (CRS JULY 2020)

Everyone seems to be focused on the patients' views on how the COVID-19 is affecting healthcare, but what about the healthcare providers' opinions? Nurses are responsible for any healthcare facility running as smoothly as it does, yet it is a rare occasion that their opinion is taken into consideration. Nurses have their own feelings about how this pandemic has affected their lives and jobs. It should be heard.

Seven nurses were asked their opinion on the COVID-19 pandemic and how they felt it was affecting the quality of care they provided. Similar to the topics discussed with patients, the nurses were asked about wearing masks, the governor and politics, media, and compliance.

Overall, every nurse was in favor of wearing the mask to prevent the spread of the virus. Even when asked about how controversial the effectiveness of the mask was, they all seemed to have the opinion that every little bit counts. Even if the mask does absolutely nothing to prevent the spread of the virus, it is not hurting anything to wear one. So, you might as well wear one just in case it does help prevent the spread. One nurse felt more strongly than other nurses about wearing the masks because the virus had affected her personally. She had previously had the virus and her mother had passed away from it. They also seemed to think that mostly the older generation was compliant, and the younger generations seemed not to care that much about wearing the mask. One nurse even said, "It's like they think they are indestructible, and their actions do not affect others."

When the governor and politics were discussed, the conversation shifted to a perspective not considered by most. Like the patients previously interviewed, the nurses also thought that the governor had done a great job at first but was now "spiraling out of control." However, they also stated that every politician seemed to be between a rock and a hard place. They said it probably had a lot to do with the populations' general opinions on political parties and personal beliefs for each politician. "You will always have those people that do the exact opposite of what the governor or president says just because they don't like them, even if it is the best thing for society to do," says one of the nurses. They also said that the media played a large role in the compliance of others. The nurses seemed to think that there is so much false information out there and it is making it difficult for people to determine what the right or wrong thing to do is. "I think the media really needs to filter what they share with the public. They need to share information that is proven to be factual and not just anything that agrees with that news source's particular opinion in the situation. It isn't doing anything to help the situation."

Overall, the discussion with the nurses was fairly productive in gaining insight from a healthcare provider's prospective on COVID-19. All seemed to be in favor of taking the necessary precautions to prevent the spread of the virus. The biggest agreement was that this ongoing battle will not come to an end until everyone has complied with the precautionary measures put in place or a vaccine is developed. However, they do not believe that will occur anytime soon and are ready for all of this to be over so they can return to their normal lives and do their jobs the way they did before COVID wrecked the nation.

It was surprising to me that few of the nurses had been asked their opinion on the pandemic. After all, nurses are right in the middle of the whole thing and the very reason that the healthcare system is able to run as well as it does. It made me realize that not everyone values nurses in the way that I do and often their opinions and ideals get overlooked. As a future physician, this made me want to incorporate my nurses' views in my practice more and take into consideration how they feel. As the old saying goes, "nurses will either make or break a doctor." Similar to the saying "happy wife, happy life," happy nurses can provide a happy medical practice. Also, why not get the opinion of someone that is on the inside of any situation? No one likes it when "big suits" make the rules when they have never actually worked in healthcare. This situation is no different.

PEOPLE ARE DYING. THAT'S NOT POLITICAL CIERRA WOODCOCK (CRS JULY 2021)

In the midst of perhaps the biggest crisis sweeping the nation, COVID-19, there are a variety of responses to the protocols put in place to prevent the spread of the virus. With the patient demographic primarily being the elderly population, a number of topics came up for discussion when the topic of masks was brought up. These topics included the governor mandating mandatory mask wearing, the shutdown of the economy, younger generations, and the media.

Patients stated their opinions on the governor, the most common response being that they agreed with his efforts in the beginning, but they are now starting to feel that he is getting out of control. They stated that the shutdown of the economy had a major impact on not only their social lives, but their health. Many patients said that their inability to be out and about had affected their physical health and mental health. Many patients reported that their eating habits were poorer than before and had exercised less than before the shutdown had occurred. They also reported that their mental health had declined, saying that lack of stimulation or activity caused them to feel down and like nothing really mattered. These statements corresponded with their physical exams and blood work, many having gained weight, having higher A1C levels, and higher LDL and triglyceride counts.

As far as wearing the mask goes, all of the patients seemed to be compliant with the regulations put in place. Although many said that the masks made it harder for them to breathe and experienced feelings of suffocation, they understood that it had to be done to prevent the spread of the virus so society could return to normal. However, there was one major frustration that I noticed that almost all patients felt about having to wear a mask. They were frustrated that they were doing their part in society by wearing the mask to protect themselves and others, but the younger generation seemed to be unconcerned and noncompliant with the masks. It was not necessarily the fact that the younger generation did not want to wear the masks, but it made them feel that the younger generation did not care about the lives of the elderly or the effects that the virus could have on them. One patient even said, "It is so frustrating to see the younger generation not doing their part. It is almost as if they think they are invincible. They may be, who knows? But we (the elderly) are not. They have no respect for our lives or authority." She went on to state that it was because children were raised to think the world revolves around them and that the rules do not apply to them. Others were even frustrated by the fact that people think it is a political scandal. "People are dying. That's not political," he said. All in all the response to wearing masks was fairly positive. All patients seemed to care about putting others at risk and how to prevent the spread of the virus.

I went into this with the preconceived thought that the elderly were the ones being least compliant and that most of them hated wearing the masks. I then saw that the elderly were not the problem, but my generation. As someone that has seen the havoc that the virus can wreak, first-hand, it made me want to be a bigger influence on my peers in being compliant with the mask regulations. As far as being a future physician goes, it made me realize that the problem does not always lie where you assume. So, it is important to keep an open mind when going into any situation, especially when dealing with a patient.

THE BUSY MOM
KENNEDY BREEDING (PRE-MATRIC JUNE 2020)

When I walked into the exam room to meet Ms. L, I quickly noticed how jittery she was. The 44 year old woman was sitting on the edge of her seat with her foot constantly tapping. This restless disposition was so apparent that I assumed she was visiting the clinic for serious lab results or something dire. However, I was surprised to learn that she simply came in for a checkup after being prescribed new medication. Upon interviewing her, I find out that as a single mother of two teenagers, Ms. L is only not used to sitting still for long periods of time.

"We are a very sporty family", she said matter of factly. Being sure to not waste any time, she went on to explain that her daughter, age 14 plays basketball and softball and her son, age 18, plays basketball and baseball. This usually keeps her schedule constantly packed with games, practices and team meetings. However, her spring season was considerably unoccupied as COVID-19 had not only cancelled all of spring sports, but also the busy graduating activities both of her children were looking forward to as a graduating high schooler and middle schooler.

Despite the fact that both of her children had to miss an entire sports season, school dances, and graduations, she remains positive about the situation. "It's something he'll definitely remember!" she comments while explaining how her son's drive through High School graduation worked.

I feel as if it was this optimism that led Ms. L to her job working with government assistance programs. "It's got its perks," she explained pondering her career. "It's so fulfilling being able to help others in need."

Presently Ms. L's schedule is returning to its pre-COVID hectic pace. Her daughter's travel softball team is beginning to practice and play games together again and her son is preparing to move out of state to play baseball at the collegiate level. Ms. L says that despite the distance, she is going to try to go to as many of his games as she can. This doesn't surprise me. Though I had only met Ms. L moments before, it was easy to see that a busy schedule hasn't kept her from her kids in the past.

Looking to the future, Ms. L wants to travel more. She is currently planning a beach vacation for her family. "I love the beach", she says with a smile. Ms. L also hopes to continue to travel after retirement. "I want to go to places I've never seen before." She says excitedly. As I left the exam room, there wasn't a doubt in my mind that Ms. L would do all she had set out to do. The jittery patient has had plenty of practice using her time to the fullest and I had a feeling that wouldn't change anytime soon.

HELPING OTHERS WHILE STAYING SAFE
MICHELE BREZINSKI MD, COMMUNITY PRACTICE

I hadn't planned on being pregnant in the middle of a pandemic. Of course, when I set out to have a sibling for my son, I hadn't planned on months upon months of labs, ultrasounds, failed procedures and bad news. When I learned I was pregnant at the end of January, it truly was a gift from above.

Then came COVID, and everything changed. I was working full time evenings and weekends in a hospital-based urgent care. It was a busy, chaotic, practice where I often saw 5-8 patients an hour. Although I wasn't a fan of the long commute, I liked my employer, my staff and the facility where I worked and most importantly, I had near total control over my schedule. When the virus first started to really make news in mid-February, I talked to my OB, who recommended wearing a mask and gloves for every patient. As the virus spread, my OB added additional protective recommendations. At 42, I was a high-risk pregnancy with nearly zero chance of another biological child if I fell ill with COVID. Our hospital administration was not willing to allow me access to PPE (even now you can only have an N95 if intubating or doing an aerosol generating procedure), and I suddenly found myself off work.

In a heartbeat, I went from being on the front lines to wondering how I was going to support myself and my son. I was fortunate to have credentialed to do telehealth several years previously, so I found myself logging in any chance I had. For those who've never practiced telemedicine, there's a bit of a learning curve, helping patients to direct phone cameras into their throats and trying to assess rashes in 2D with suboptimal lighting. As the pandemic spread, telemedicine was flooded with COVID cases and patients who were too afraid to go to their local health care facility.

I was still practicing mostly urgent care, however the nature of my practice, and the pace of it, had changed dramatically. Despite the dramatic reduction in compensation, I soon found that the change wasn't all bad. The perpetual exhaustion from working till midnight and getting up with my son before 5am gradually disappeared. The heartburn and bloating that had been my constant companions for the last six months resolved as I started to eat meals all in one sitting, instead of a bite or two between patients over a several hour time window. Despite typical pregnancy symptoms, I started to feel more like myself than I had in many years.

As it becomes clear that this pandemic isn't going to ease significantly over the next 6-12 months, I've begun to reflect on where my career in medicine will go from here. I know I don't enjoy traditional outpatient clinic practice and my schedule as a hospitalist wasn't compatible with life as a parent. As a single mom of a two year old boy and a soon to be newborn, the thought of going back to acute care medicine is terrifying. My access to PPE will still be limited, and I will be facing the potential of bringing this illness home to my children, or becoming ill myself and unable to care for them, maybe forever. I chose medicine out of a desire to help others, yet this pandemic has taught me that I must find a way to serve without risking the safety of my family. I have learned much about my profession and the health system I work in over the last two months, yet the most precious lessons have nothing – and everything – to do with being a physician. I've learned to honor my own health and my personal values. I finally understand that I can care for others without sacrificing that which I hold most dear. I don't yet know where my path goes from here, but that's okay. Nothing is certain anymore. Nothing except love.

I CAN'T SHAKE YOUR HAND
TATE BURRIS (CRS JULY 2020)

We are all currently faced with an incredible challenge that nobody thought they would ever be faced with in their lifetime, we are currently living through a global pandemic. COVID-19 has caught everyone by surprise and has changed the way we go about so many different things in our lives. One thing that has been affected very heavily is how we supply healthcare. In order to minimize the spread of the virus, healthcare workers are having to change the way they do their job. An opening handshake has been traded for a hello and awkward stares, being close to your patient has turned into being no less than six feet apart until absolutely necessary, and most prominently, a friendly smile has been traded for a mask. At first glance you wouldn't think that wearing a mask would affect the doctor patient relationship that much, I mean doctors wear masks all the time for some procedures. That is correct but for a normal visit wearing a mask makes things the tiniest bit more difficult. People who are already hard to verbally understand become even more difficult do to the muffled sound of your voice, but what I have seen the most is that it is now so hard to express and pick up nonverbal cues. You can no longer see a person's smile or frown or grimace. And subsequently, as a physician you now must find a way to show your happiness besides a smile, and you must now find a new way to let the patient know you are listening by other ways besides the intent look on your face. The masks are important to stopping the spread of the virus, and even though the masks have made things more difficult, they are definitely not impossible. If it is hard to hear someone wearing a mask, we learn to speak louder, if it's hard to show facial expressions to a patient to let them know that you are listening and want the best for them, you learn different ways of showing it. Throughout this time physicians have learned how to adapt to these crazy times we live and still do the important job that they do even if it might look a little different from what it used to look like.

In looking at my shadowing experiences from this past week I was very pleasantly surprised how smoothly everything was run despite the restrictions and protocols due to COVID-19. Besides the masks and no touching, it felt just like business as usual. Now I am sure this is not how it has been the whole time. Physicians have had plenty of time to adjust their style and how they go about practicing medicine until now. In looking at them now it seems almost like they have been practicing this way their entire life. Does that mean that everything is perfect, of course not. It is still difficult for them to not shake someone's hand, or give them a hug when they are happy from good news. They have had to change the way that they express their emotions to the patient, and sometimes that can be difficult, but as a whole from the doctors I have seen this week, they have been able to adapt very easily.

SIX FEET APART
TATE BURRIS (CRS JULY 2020)

Social distancing has become a pivotal part of today's society. We all must be diligent in making sure that we remain six feet apart from other people to help decrease the spread of COVID. Just like every other aspect of dealing with COVID, social distancing has changed the way that physicians practice medicine. Because you must keep your distance, you can no longer shake someone's hand as you walk in the room. You can no longer sit next to the patient and put your hand on their shoulder as a sign that you understand what they are struggling with and that you care about them. Because of COVID, these interactions have been traded for six feet of distance and awkward stares. Physicians are searching for new ways to express that they are emotionally invested with this patient, but there is just no better way than a hug or a hand on the shoulder. Sitting on the other side of the room making eye contact and nodding your head up and down just doesn't have the same affect. Now this is not to say that these other methods are ineffective by any means, it is just that nothing will be as effective as human contact. Health care continues to change during this pandemic, and we may never get back to the way things used to be, which could be both a good and a bad thing. At least we are seeing that there are different ways to practice medicine that are still effective and keep people as safe as possible, but we have also limited the patient physician interaction which is both one of the most important, and most rewarding parts of the job. Nothing feels better than a patient you have been seeing for years walking into an appointment telling you that he hasn't felt that good in years and giving you a hug. It really makes you feel like you made a difference, and even though you can still keep that feeling without the physical contact, it just isn't as personal.

From my personal experiences, I think that physicians have done a great job adapting to all of the regulations of social distancing. It has been hard for them, because for years they have done things a certain way and then almost overnight they had to change. For them it is almost first nature to walk into a room and immediately shake the patient's hand, but physicians are having to catch themselves. They walk in and immediately pull their hands from their pockets and go to reach out until they remember that they can't do that and pull back. Through personal observation, even though they have had to change all these little things that they do, the quality of their work has not dropped. These physicians realize that this is the world we live in now, and they can either be upset by it, or learn how to adapt and keep providing high quality care in different ways. It is important that everybody takes note from physicians when it comes to social distancing. If everybody decided that even though it might be hard and would make you change the ways you do certain things, that if we all took social distancing serious this virus would be gone sooner rather than later.

TELEMEDICINE IS ADVANTAGEOUS
SUMMER SPARKS (CRS JULY 2020)

The COVID-19 pandemic has been extremely challenging for all professionals to feel as though they can adequately perform their duties. For health care professionals specifically, COVID-19 has changed the way these professionals interact and effectively treat their patients. At the beginning of the pandemic, many outpatient health care facilities closed entirely, leaving many patients without access to routine health care. Many facilities dramatically changed their methods for seeing patients. Fortunately, these facilities transitioned to telemedicine in order to have some contact with patients and/or developed other strategies to see patients safely.

Telemedicine has proven to be extremely advantageous. Many patients seem to prefer the convenient video calls to in person visits. It has been especially useful for those with busy schedules and who may have difficulty finding the time to visit a health care facility. Telemedicine is also helpful to many patients who consider in-person office visits inaccessible such as patients who struggle with social anxiety or a physical illness making travel difficult. It is also helpful to those who may not have transportation to the facility. There have been some issues, however, with health care facilities putting full reliance on telemedicine. Often, elderly patients have difficulty utilizing the technology required for telemedicine. Sometimes, especially in rural communities, the internet connection is not always optimal for seeing one's physician over video call. This makes communication between patient and physician less effective. Now, many facilities are attempting to do some in-person visits and some telemedicine visits. This poses a problem for many physicians. Often, many office visits take longer than anticipated. This will cause the physician to get behind on televisits. Occasionally, the patient will log onto the video call application at the time of his or her appointment and the physician will not be available. This confusion sometimes causes the patient to disconnect the application thinking it is not working properly.

Overall, other precautions also have some pros and cons. Social distancing and mask-wearing make in-office visits seem impersonal. Patients have a more difficult time conveying their emotional states to their physicians because they are limited on the nonverbal gestures they can use. They also feel as though they cannot show gratitude to their physicians and the physician's staff as easily without smiling. Conversely, these safety precautions, although inconvenient, ensures the patients' safety if they come in for a visit. Knowing that a facility is following safety regulations assures patients that they will be protected as much as possible from COVID-19 while in the facility. Physicians' are also being protected from the virus because patients must answer screening questions and have their temperatures taken prior to entering the facility.

In the future, I believe that telemedicine will be commonly utilized in most health care facilities. Unfortunately, COVID-19 forced many facilities to begin using telemedicine before being properly trained. It is fortunate that we, as a society, have had the ability to use telemedicine during this time. Without it, many patients would have been without medicine refills or essential medical counseling. As insurance companies begin to offer reimbursement, physicians will be able to use telemedicine for many non-essential visits. This is useful because physicians will be able to allocate more time to patients who require more time and attention during in-office visits. I also think that as society is learning to take precautions to mitigate the effects of COVID-19, patients will also be protected from other contagious illnesses by employing the same infection control measures.

HURTING TO HEAL
REBECCA BOLLINGER (MS 3 OCTOBER 2020)

The unknown, the uncertainty, the unclear expectations: the prodrome of the Coronavirus for me. When I first heard about this virus spreading, I dusted off the vague memory of the mention of a virus named "corona" two years prior, located somewhere in the midst of all the other information your first year of medical school drowns you in. It had seemed miniscule and unimportant at the time, like a book your grandma let you borrow years ago in your bookcase that you shoved among fifty others that you have yet to read. Now, though, this book had pulled itself off the shelf and demanded the world read it. I wouldn't have believed then if someone of authority and intelligence had told me that this coronavirus we were studying would come like a tsunami, interrupting our third year of medical school, overwhelming the doctors and residents that we had grown to respect and love, ravaging the lives of many of us, and bringing with it a fear we have never experienced and so much uncertainty about what tomorrow would hold.

From afar, I watched with foggy eyes and ignorant, distant concern as the infectious wave called Coronavirus made its name halfway across the world. I remember feeling immunity, nonchalance, carelessness as we often do when we have lived our whole lives with no life-threatening entity ever coming close to knocking at our door. Even after hearing it was in our country I continued, planning out my fourth year of medical school meticulously, ensuring that I had considered all options and had everything exactly where it best fit. After somewhere between 8 and 15 drafts of the schedule, I was satisfied. My remaining requirements to ensure I would have MD after my name were finally on paper, and I could breathe, knowing that I was in complete control of my methodically planned out future.

The first of the virus in my life came in the form of patient concern. I remember this sweet elderly lady coming in for a weeklong history of insomnia due to excessive worry about this Coronavirus. With fear evident on her face, she recited some lines from the news that had obviously consumed her television lately. I watched as the doctor I was working with patted her knee and with every good and caring intention reassured her that we were all safe. This virus was nothing more that the flu. I nodded in confidence alongside her.

Soon after came the delays, the changes in our busy third year clinical schedule which we all hoped would not interfere with our carefully thought out, prayed over, fought for, lottery-determined fourth year blueprints. Our lives as students up to this point had been planned out years in advance, the expectations laid out clearly- our exact tasks to complete, their due dates, as well as the consequences for not fulfilling the requirements. To get where we are now means we have thrived under those clear directions. And now, looking at the faces of our leadership on the screen of our laptops, we hear the words, "If you are on clinical rotation right now, go home. We do not know when you will return or what the days ahead hold." This virus was now powerful enough to halt our schedules filled with long and demanding days, and it was finally real to me.

I, along with my 161 fellow classmates, entered the medical field because of our overly-cliché interview response but truly genuine desire to help people. We chose the medical profession so we can be there with people in their most vulnerable times to offer our knowledge and our capabilities in order to relieve some of the suffering they experience. In this great time of suffering that had come, we suddenly found ourselves at home- with no one to comfort and no one to help but ourselves. The largest health crisis we had ever seen combined with our fresh passion to help was a recipe for frustration. I realize now, though, that our fresh, overly ambitious desire to serve the sick and hurting could be dangerous in its naïve third-year-of-med-school form that it currently exists.

Along with frustration, maybe even contradictory to it, I felt relief. As the realness of this virus and the devastating war it could rage on the lining of lungs and the cytokine storm it could initiate in our bodies came to be understood, I felt myself being relieved to be on this side of my Doctor of Medicine Degree. I wanted to help and serve, but the weight of the potential consequences of working as an Essential Employee in a hospital, being exposed to a potentially deadly disease, was something I had rarely considered until this time. Those on the other side of their degree were dutifully and self-sacrificially putting themselves at risk every day in order to keep the Oath they made to the good of mankind. While half of me craved to be there, the other half clung tightly to the safety of my self-quarantine.

While these feelings swirled around together in the steaming pot of my brain, which was boiling over right in front of me, I noticed something else simmering on the backburner. It was my concern about my educational success as a medical student. I was, in fact, still in the middle of a clerkship- and not just any. I was in the middle of the clerkship in the field that I want to pursue. This meant that poor performance on my upcoming shelf exam could be detrimental to reaching my professional goals (or at least it felt this way at the time).

How do you study the material that you will use to care for patients two years from now when a disease with the capability to kill is travelling around your very own country, your very own state, and now your very own city? When you have an exam in three days and someone who lives ten minutes from you tests positive, how do you keep your head in books? Usually my exams are my biggest tsunamis, but I realized then that they are safe little tsunamis: predictable, maybe damaging, but definitely not life threatening. I felt like a school kid living in an unsafe situation at home and still being expected to practice my times-tables every night. How do you focus on the math homework on your table when your survival is on the table right beside it?

As we all press on with our lives during the slow passing of quarantine time, I am beginning to believe that though this virus brings the impossibility of focusing enough to learn the screening guidelines for hyperlipidemia, it brings with it more vital lessons. It is true that the feelings the Coronavirus has evoked in us and the tragedy that it has caused for many people will forever affect us. The schedules that have been destroyed, the monumental life events that have been cancelled, the overwhelming anxiety that inhibits our sleep, the people whom we have lost, the suffering in isolation, the political dramatics, the financial struggles, and the continued uncertainty of when life will return to normal or if it ever will- these things are ours to live with. And these things hurt.

I believe, though, that our hurting can pave the way for healing to occur. Might this virus that has infected the world and our communities leave us with resistance to some other of life's diseases and bring healing to the ones that already infect us? Maybe its wildness will bring us a humility as we realize our smallness in this world, washing away our pride and false sense of control. It may push us to treasure those people in our lives more than the things we possess as we realize the frailty of human life. Might it press us into a place of self-reflection, allowing us to learn more about ourselves as we face our own minds? As it takes away the day-to-day busyness, it may grant us time to admire the little things in life. Putting us worldwide in the same boat, might it give us a feeling of oneness as a human race? Maybe it will strip us of our own daily self-centered preoccupations and give us some perspective and compassion. I believe the immense wave of uncertainty that has washed over us during this time could carry our other uncertainties away with it as it goes, leaving us with more certainty- about who we are, what is important, and how we want to move forward.

My fourth year schedule, though it has been torn, is re-constructible. I know that not all that this virus has destroyed is re-constructible, though. I realize that this disease is a devastation, and I could never begin to understand the extent of that devastation in all individual lives affected. As this pandemic has taught us, though, we only have so much time on this earth, so why not allow this inevitable tsunami to power our healing?

MASKS ARE A MINOR INCONVENIENCE
TATE BURRIS (CRS JULY 2020)

The more and more that I shadow during this strange time, the more I realize that things in the clinical setting really haven't changed as much as I thought they would have during this pandemic. Of course, there are little changes here and there, and everyone wearing masks is still a significant difference, but as a whole, the way that the clinic works is not very different than it was before COVID. Besides the fact that there a far less walk in visits every day, the number of established patient visits only saw a small decline. And as it relates to the doctor patient interactions, sure there was no handshake at the start, but everything else about the visit was done the exact same way it would have been done before the COVID pandemic. They still asked all the same questions, and did all the same physical exams, even the ones that required the doctor to put their hands on the patients, they just had to make sure that their hands were clean, which they had to do in the first place. Surprisingly there was very little telemedicine done. In a time where we are encouraged to keep contact with other people to a minimum, I expected there to be an increase in the amount of care given over the phone, but still the vast majority of patients were seen in office. Dr. M even said that, "I have to see them in person, it's hard to trust what you can't see right in front of you." Even in this time of social distancing and caution, at eye level health care hasn't really changed that much, sure some of the logistics and protocols have changed, but at the patient physician level, not much has changed.

I really enjoyed seeing how everything worked in a clinical setting during this time of pandemic. But in all honesty, I expected my experience to be incredibly different than any of my shadowing experiences so far, but that really wasn't the case. Besides having to wear a mask while in the rooms, I really didn't feel like much was different. While you were there in the clinic, you didn't think about COVID. You had a patient, and it was your job to help them feel better no matter what, and in that sense, it was business as usual. People still came into the office, there was still contact between the doctor and the patient, the only difference was that everyone was wearing a mask, which at the end of the day is only a minor inconvenience. Now of course everyone is very cautious, and the numbers of patients coming in is decreased, which definitely affects the workplace in some way, but not nearly as much as I thought it was going to.

STARTING MEDICAL SCHOOL DURING A PANDEMIC
EMMA DOYLE (PRE-MATRIC JUNE 2020)

When I pictured myself in medical school, I had always seen myself precepting in a busy practice, meeting patients all day and trying to absorb as much information as I can. Then, in March of my last year of undergraduate work, COVID-19 had become such a threat that schools, businesses, and even healthcare facilities were shuttered everywhere. Starting medical school began to take on an entirely new shape as innovation in healthcare was accelerated at incredible speeds. I have nearly completed my pre-matriculation program now, and I have certainly noticed radical changes in the way care is administered to patients in light of the pandemic.

For the past three weeks, I have shadowed a great deal in a rural health clinic in Western Kentucky. Although the physician I shadowed sees about thirty patients each day, only about two or three of those have been in-person visits. The other appointments have been changed to either video or telephone visits, depending on the patients' needs or preferences. As a result, most of my time has been spent in the doctor's office, unable to see the patients with which the physician was speaking. Although telehealth offers convenience and safety, some telehealth visits prove to be a wasteful. In several cases, the physician was unable to make a diagnosis of a condition without an in-person physical exam. For example, one woman complained of having a rash on the back of her neck, which the poor resolution of the video conference prevented the physician from seeing well enough to identify. In this sort of case, patients are asked to call the receptionist to make an in-person appointment for a later date. This sort of gap between the tele-visit and the more fruitful in-person visit could delay the delivery of care to patients, possibly allowing their conditions to get worse.

Whether in-person or not, almost every conversation between patient and physician includes some mention of the virus or the pandemic. Patients often mention that wearing a mask causes them anxiety or makes breathing difficult. Physicians will often ask their patients how they are handling life since the pandemic began, either to make conversation or to assess their emotional wellbeing.

Everyone in the healthcare facility must now wear a mask while they are in the building. Healthcare workers are provided masks, and patients who do not have a mask are provided one when they enter. The mask offers a bit of peace of mind that the spread of the virus is slowed in the healthcare facility, but the mask also proves a barrier to expressing emotions that are crucial in patient-physician interaction. Each must rely on the other's expression in their eyes since smiles, frowns, or grimaces are completely covered. I have not asked a physician how they feel about this, but while I have spoken to patients, I have noticed myself nodding or shaking my head more fervently to get a point across, supplementing the concealment of my mouth. The physician mask also serves as a distraction for patient and physician. Many patients continually adjust their mask throughout the visit. While adjusting the mask, the patient seems less concerned with what the physician is saying while the physician's eyes are drawn to the mask and away from the patient.

Many doctors have taken note that their patients' general health has deteriorated since social distancing guidelines and closures began. Patients have been forced to stay in their homes for several weeks with less access to nutritious foods and exercise. As a result, physicians note that their patients have increased incidence of anxiety and depression, high blood pressure, and weight gain in the last several months. The incidence of weight gain even has a name among several health professionals that I have shadowed: the "COVID-15." Although patients are kept safe from the virus by staying at home more often, their long-term health may be worse.

Perhaps the one most understated changes in the wake of the COVID-19 pandemic has been a physical distancing between patient and physician in the exam room. When a patient comes for a first visit with a new doctor, the pair no longer shake hands in greeting. Introductions feel more awkward as a result of losing the widely held custom; no one in the exam room really knows how to begin a visit anymore. Some physicians I have shadowed have resorted to waving to their patients when entering the exam room, which seems to give the relationship a more casual tone from the onset. As an alternative to waving, I followed an OB/GYN that opted to "air" shake hands with her new patients from a distance, which initiated a new doctor/patient relationship with a lighthearted and humorous tone. Handshakes are not the only social physical contact a physician has lost. COVID-19 has also stopped physicians from touching their patients to console them. I would not have noticed this except for seeing a patient visit a family physician shortly after learning that she had stage three breast cancer. When the doctor and I entered the exam room, the patient was crying alone on the exam table. Under normal circumstances, the physician may have touched her patient's shoulder or even embraced her patient to console her. As with any other patient, though, considerations regarding the spread of COVID-19 had to be taken, and so the physician could not touch her patient more than was necessary for her examination. Instead, the physician could only offer a sympathetic expression in her eyes through the emotional barrier of a face shield and mask. For anyone feeling this kind of fear, having a care provider offer you sympathy from a physical distance might not feel like sympathy at all.

As my peers and I are entering medical school, the physicians we learn from have told us often that healthcare will soon be radically different from what they have been taught; they expect the COVID-19 pandemic to mean to healthcare what 9/11 meant for airlines. Virtually nothing will be the same. Most doctors expect telehealth to remain prevalent, and many expect mental health to go through a substantial slump. Depending on how quickly a vaccine or treatment is made, physical distancing may continue for a long time. No matter the results, it seems that upcoming medical students like me will have to face an uncertain future in healthcare, and we will have to be flexible to grow into a field that is changing before our eyes.

IT HASN'T STOPPED
LAUREN TROUT (CRS JULY 2022)

It has been over two years and the fear is still lingering. Every sore throat, every cough, every raised temperature. It has to be COVID. The urgent care was overrun with COVID tests. One after another after another. The symptoms aren't near as bad and the mortality rate is down, but yet several are still mortified

BARRIERS TO HUMAN CONNECTION
MARIA SHIELDS (PRE-MATRIC JUNE 2020)

Faces garnished with masks and shield, the provider enters the patient room. As if in their own separate bubbles, they begin their long-awaited conversation. Although spoken language is transmitted, much is lost during the exchange. Perhaps the patient speaks of their success in weight loss or smoking cessation - hidden remains the joy and smile of their provider tucked behind thick woven cloth. These barriers to infectious disease filter out much more than microscopic organisms; they filter the very human connection upon which we all rely in our daily interactions.

Joy and fear, among other emotions, become muddled in the age of COVID-19. A woman has received news that her cancer has returned - hidden remains the sadness etched across her once beaming smile. A young mother has learned that she has finally conceived after years of IVF - hidden remains the newly found smile she struggled to find for years. This language without spoken words provides incredible opportunity to connect with our fellow human beings. Often unconscious and one of the rawest forms of communication, facial expression is a crucial part of understanding someone's comfort and connection to the world around them. Face masks introduce the opportunity for patients to sense a lack of empathy from the same providers from which they expect and deserve understanding.

The face mask has the power to morph some of the nation's most compassionate physicians into a vessel of knowledge from whom a patient no longer senses empathy. We undoubtedly have faces masks to thank for the slowed spread of infectious diseases and preservation of health for many. But have we also considered that the same masks that may preserve our physical health, may also be harmful for our mental health and the health outcomes of our patients? The face mask is now a double-edged sword with the power to both defend and harm.

As medical students, we often rely heavily upon the joy and fear our patients exude. Similarly, our patients rely upon us to celebrate their victories and mourn in their losses. A smile has the power to alleviate fear, demonstrate shared joy, or even provide hope in the midst of bad news. These reactions and responses void of words, must now be explicitly communicated. Face masks necessitate the need for more - more words, more explanation, and more questions - while allowing us to give less to our patients. This relentless cycle of supply and demand is complicated by the growing expectations of the U.S. healthcare system at large where productivity and time are valued treasures. In a new world where more is expected from the healthcare system, the healthcare providers that comprise it are struggling more than ever to connect to their patients and provide compassionate healthcare. In a time where we all need more support and connection, we face unprecedented barriers to human connection.

BATTLE RASH
CAITLAN JONES (CRS JULY 2020)

COVID-19 has shaken the world and doesn't seem to stop wreaking havoc anytime soon. While scientist and researchers are scrambling to create and ensure a safe and effective vaccine, common folk are puzzled. Between science presenting us with new discoveries that may even contradict what we were told last week, to a heated political climate, to the flooding of "corona" articles on Facebook, people are confused on what to believe. And yet it isn't just the 35-year-old who is losing business every day or the 65-year-old grandmother fearing for her life that are affected, but its children as well. We often overlook children and how trauma affects them. They are resilient we say, as we assume that they will be alright because we have bigger fish to fry than stacking Legos. And yet, I would like to take a moment to examine how COVID-19 has and will affect children of all ages. I find no better way to do this than to look at a smiley face child-sized mask.

Little Ben came into the office wound up and afraid of the doctor. A young kid, but old enough that he was given a mask to wear in the office. As we looked at his severe allergic reaction that literally covered his body, I noticed how pure of a moment it was. His mother had blown up a medical glove with air so he would stay occupied and sit still while he continually called me 'that girl over there'. He had probably never been to the doctor with a student in the room. He informed me that he had a battle-rash instead of a battle scar, and all the while that smiley face-mask remained unused on the counter. At that moment, the last thing I wanted was for him to have to put the mask on. I could see his teeth when he giggled and I could understand his broken, slurred toddler talk. Nevertheless, as he was getting ready to leave the office after the physician placed an order for some medicine, his mom had him put the mask on. It took a lot of convincing as his little brain couldn't wrap itself around the idea in the first place. It wasn't long though that his tiny nose and mouth were covered and the spread of germs was decreased. Children are as confused as we adults are. They don't understand why they must wear a mask and have a rough time leaving it alone. I've seen kiddos pull them down, wear them over their eyes and use them to avoid making connections with those around them. Our children are hurting, our teenagers are hurting. If they must also wear a mask, then their thoughts and concerns must also be validated. We must remember that they too are affected by this mess of a pandemic, but also that they are, after all, kids. We must keep them safe but we must also not rob them of a childhood either.

EXPRESSING COMPASSION BEHIND THE MASK
HANNAH MARSHALL (CRS JULY 2020)

In any healthcare setting, masks can present a multitude of issues. One of the most basic forms of communication stems from non-verbal cues such as facial expressions. In medicine, facial expressions are often used to express a feeling of understanding or empathy, and masks seem to have posed an issue for this in some practices. Currently in almost all practice settings masks are required for the patient and for the provider and staff and occasionally face visors and other forms of PPE are also required. It is evident that the amount of necessary caution can cause communication issues. Alongside masks, many practices have resorted to using tele-health to communicate or to be an alternative to an in-person visit.

With all the potential complications that can arise from tele-health as well as wearing masks, I observed no large differences in operations at the community health clinic. They had screeners that asked a variety of questions to rule out COVID as well as a temperature screen. The screener ensured the patient was wearing a mask. It was evident that many patients did not enjoy the masks, however many were willing to wear them and understood the importance of the mask.

Dr. G did not do any tele-health visits, but from talking with the nurses, the office did do tele-health if the patient preferred it. He also seemed to adapt well to overcome the obstacle of non-verbal communication by expressing to the patient his feelings and emotions verbally rather than facially. Dr. G was not extremely strict with the masks, he stated that if a patient was extremely uncomfortable wearing a mask, he would allow them to take it off during their visit.

When talking with the patients I asked if any had felt that COVID placed an inconvenience in their ability to obtain healthcare recently. Many stated that they had no issues with Dr. G, as his practice never slowed down, and generally had no issues wearing a mask. Many expressed that they felt safer wearing masks out and were glad that there was at least something they could do to prevent the spread of COVID.

Personally, I was surprised with how compliant the patients were with the masks. In my personal experience many people are non-compliant with masks and seem to have issues with wearing them. The population that Dr. G sees is typically an older population, and many of his patients act out of fear when wearing the masks. They are more concerned with their health and the consequences of COVID rather than the mask being uncomfortable or causing an inconvenience.

Dr. G did not do any tele-health when I was with him this week; however, next week I hope to sit in with his nurse practitioner and watch some tele-health visits. Many patients seemed to prefer in-person visits due to age and lack of technology. I would be curious to see what number of his patients were physically able to do tele-health and which weren't able.

FACIAL EXPRESSIONS ARE JUST AS IMPORTANT AS WORDS
BLAKE EDMONSON (PRE-MATRIC JUNE 2020)

Historically, the face mask has been seen as a sign of a serious medical situation, such as infectious disease or surgery. Its use was limited in the medical field but has always served as a safety precaution. However, instances of plagues or epidemics have brought forth more common usages for the face mask. COVID-19 specifically has created a widespread need for face masks for everyday use to prevent further spread. The need grew so rapidly that there was even a shortage of face masks available in the first weeks of the spread of the virus. The face mask has since become an integral part of every individual's life. Requirements for a face mask have been implemented in almost every form of society, not just in the medical field. The vast usage has allowed the face mask to become part of normality in our society. It used to be viewed as a negative sign but has now become a sign of activism in the awareness of the epidemic.

Personally, the face mask has become a hindrance. Over the past three weeks, I have had the privilege to shadow physicians and interview patients. However, the face mask has greatly influenced the overall impact of such activities. Facial expressions are just as revealing as the actual words spoken when conversing with a patient. Often, I rely on these expressions to truly understand the overall mood or tone of a person. The face mask has hindered my ability to do so. The conversations I have been able to have were still impactful in nature but were diminished in their intensity. I have still been able to listen and observe the life stories and medical histories of many patients, but it has been a struggle to fully understand the severity and sincerity in such stories. I personally struggle with some minor hearing loss in both of my ears with my right ear being more affected than the left. I often catch myself reading lips or at least following along with lips to understand what is being said. The prevalence of face masks in our society has hindered my ability to understand many individuals. I catch myself having to ask people to repeat things several times or have them speak louder. This itself slows down the progression of conversation and often arouses annoyances with some individuals.

Overall, the face mask has posed a new factor in the everyday life of most citizens. While seen as a positive way to contribute to the prevention of the spread of the virus, many people have come to resent the face mask. Some even believe it does not have an effect on preventing further spread. Either way, the face mask will continue to a part of our lives as it has become an integral part of functioning society.

MASKING OUR SMILE
CAITLAN JONES (CRS JULY 2020)

A Smile. Oh how it warms a room, breaks the ice, and reminds us that we are in fact, human. Whether surrounded in cherry red lipstick or lacking a few teeth, a smile can connect two seemingly different people. A smile can immediately build trust, and it can spark a conversation. A smile makes the world's difference when meeting a stranger. But what happens when the smile seizes to be seen? What happens when you no longer notice gapped teeth, a nervously forced half smile, a quivering bottom lip, or the genuineness of who you're facing? While masks, surgical or otherwise, may be an important piece of personal protective equipment, it comes at a cost. It is not just covering our faces in an effort to block a virus, but it is masking our smiles too.

The health care field is engulfed in the positives and negatives of masks. On one hand they have shown to reduce the chance of transmitting a scarily unknown virus, and on the other they are complicating physician patient interactions. One of the key components to treating a patient is getting the patient to trust you, especially when they are seeing a new physician for the very first time. While the use of surgical or medical grade masks became widespread in the 1960s there are still many sectors of medicine where a mask isn't so common. Before Covid-19 a doctor, nurse, or patient wearing a cloth or surgical mask in a primary care facility was a rarity. But now, it's standard. For example, our Community

Health Center requests that all patients wear a mask upon arrival, if not they will be given one once in office. As a student observer, I quickly noticed that the small, rural practice did in fact stick to these guidelines and all provider-patient interactions involved a face covering. One notable exception was one physician's use of a plastic face shield instead of a mask. Before entering a patient's room, he explained to me that he chooses to wear a face shield so that his patients can see him. Having only been at the practice for 7 months, many of his patients were new and being able to see and recognize his face was a huge help. Family practice is deeply rooted in making personal connections and treating a family for a lifetime. The use of a see-through face shield increased personability and made it easier for patients to hear and understand the doctor's guidance.

Another sector of medicine that masks have complicated is Behavioral Health. In Psychiatry it is imperative to connect with the patient and make them feel comfortable enough to discuss their mental health. Sitting and talking with a patient in a behavioral facility is a large part of treatment. And what do you do when you discuss mental health with a patient? You sit close, stay engaged, and show them you are sincerely interested by your body language. However, the masks required by nearly all hospitals and facilities block some of that body language. It is hard to tell tone, humor, and compassion when you only hear a voice and cannot visually connect. Dr. J at the in-patient behavioral health services unit said that masks have been the hardest part of ALL the COVID-19 changes. Not the swabbing, not the social distancing, but needing to wear masks for their own and their patient's protection from a potentially deadly virus. It will be interesting to see what COVID-19 protocols stay in healthcare and what goes after the pandemic has subsided. When the threat becomes minimal, will we still wear masks every day when with patients? Or will practices weigh the pros and cons and consider not just the biological side of medicine but also the interpersonal side. Will we once again be able to see a smile?

AT LEAST I STILL GET MY DISCOUNT
CIERRA WOODCOCK (PRE-CLINICAL JULY 2022)

Mrs. AR is a 78-year-old female admitted to the hospital for hyperglycemia three days ago. From the moment I walked in, I could tell that Mrs.

AR loved to talk. She was more than willing to talk about her life, which included using her mobile device to show me an array of photos taken throughout her life.

Mrs. AR's early life began when her father, originally from Norway, came to the United States as a professional boxer. He then joined the United States Army and ended up in Dayton, Ohio, where he met her mother. They married and had her in 1944. Soon after, her family moved to Western KY, where her mother was originally from. She spent her younger life there and attended high school. She spent most of her life being a hairdresser and attending church regularly. Church became a very important part of her life and is where she met her husband, whom she has been married to for 34 years. They have a son and daughter together, two grandchildren, and one great grandchild. Before her husband retired from the coal mines, she would travel the country with him, seeing what she deems as "the best places in the U.S." Her favorite memories include going to Utah for the summer with her grandsons, and touring Mt. Zion National Park and the Grand Canyon. After her husband retired, he became a minister, and she spent the next 14 years working at a local chain restaurant because she "is a people person and loves the discounts." She spent those years heavily involving her family in church and takes great pride in how each of them has expanded on their faith in their everyday lives.

Unfortunately, Mrs. AR was laid off when restaurants shut down for COVID-19. She says although she misses working with all the people, she is not too down about it because they still let her keep her discount. She was also thankful for her somewhat forced retirement because her husband had a stroke that left him disabled and blind. She has dedicated the last two years to caring for him and spends all her time with family. When asked what she would like to see in her future, she stated "I would love nothing more than to spend the rest of my days watching my great grandson grow into a man, but I'm 78 so we'll see how far I can make it. God has truly blessed me with the most amazing life, and I intend to spend the rest of my days enjoying it." Before leaving, Mrs. AR made sure to give me what I thought was the most sincere advice I have ever received. She told me to keep looking forward to what can happen in life and always allow God to lead me in the right direction.

THE OUTDOORSY TYPE
EMMA DOYLE (PRE-MATRIC JUNE 2020)

As Dr. C shows me to her exam room, she explains that her next patient, Mr. W, has been experiencing abdominal pain. Mr. W is sitting alone in a corner chair with his hands laying in his lap with fingers interlaced. He is wearing black tennis shoes, gray shorts, and a gray cutoff tee-shirt. His arms and legs are adorned with a tapestry of tattoos of flaming human skulls and ornate lettering. Mr. W's shirt also reveals a hint of a back tattoo. His head is shaved, but he wears a long brown beard down to his belly. His demeanor is thoughtful and careful, but his distinct Western Kentucky drawl is unmistakable.

Dr. C introduces me to Mr. W and asks him to describe his pain. He tells us that a deep aching pain began just ventral to the small of his back and has radiated slowly toward his front over the course of two weeks. He says the pain was so intense on the first day that he vomited twice. The pain has been better since that time, but Mr. W still describes the feeling as "double over" pain. He can only find relief when he is able to walk and move around. Dr. C tells Mr. W that she fears he has a kidney stone, especially if the pain eases with activity, explaining that any inflammatory cause would cause the patient to feel the most pain while moving. She orders a STAT CT scan and bloodwork, asking Mr. W to return later when the results from the lab and imaging arrive.

Later in the afternoon, Mr. W returns. Dr. C is behind in her schedule, and I ask her if I should take time to talk to him while he waits. I make my way back to the exam room and reintroduce myself. I ask Mr. W if he would be willing to talk to me about his life, to which he calmly agrees. I sit in a stool opposite his seat and position myself to take some notes. I invite Mr. W to tell me about himself, and after a moment of consideration and a small sigh, he tells me that he is "pretty boring" and that there is not much to talk about. I reassure Mr. W that almost no one's life is truly boring, and I lightly encourage him to tell me about himself anyway if he can.

Mr. W begins by telling me that he has four children: a fifteen-year-old daughter, a nine-year-old daughter, a nine-year old son, and an eight-year old daughter. The children have three different mothers that they all live with now. Mr. W lives with his new girlfriend at his farm. He says the relationship has been going strong for three years now and that he has no complaints at all living with his girlfriend.

For the last fifteen years, Mr. W has worked as an underground coal miner. I ask him what the work is like, and he says with a chuckle that coal mining is not for everybody. Mr. W describes coal mining as a rough job, detailing that the mines are dark and cramped. Recently, however, Mr. W has been laid off his job at the mine. I ask him why, and Mr. W says that since the economy went bad in the midst of the COVID-19 pandemic, the mine has been struggling to turn a profit and was forced to lay off some of its most valuable workers. Mr. W is not sure when he will return to work. He mentions, however, that the extra free time has at least given him some extra time to visit with his children.

At home Mr. W runs a farm where he raises chickens and cattle. He also grows a plethora of vegetables which he lists: tomatoes, okra, potatoes, zucchini, squash, and many others. After reciting his list of crops, Mr. W is not even sure if he has mentioned everything he grows. Mr. W tells me that he must remember the growing conditions of each plant, including how much light they prefer, how much water they need, and when to plant them. I remind Mr. W that this must be no simple feat and I commend him for carrying so much expertise.

When Mr. W is not in the mines or tending to his farm, he enjoys hiking and hunting. Mr. W hunts deer, turkeys, ducks, and "everything." Every year he is able to fill his freezer with meat from hunting and eats the meat all throughout the winter. Mr. W has even begun to take his children out on hunting expeditions and smiles around his mask when he mentions how much the five of them love to hunt together. Mr. W describes himself as an "outdoorsy kind of guy," mentioning that he likes to keep himself busy and that he is not one for watching television.

From what he tells me, Mr. W seems to genuinely enjoy his life, despite his belief that it is uninteresting. He tells me he is happy living with his girlfriend on their hillside home, and that he would not have his life be any different.

I thank Mr. W for his time, and I promise an accurate story to be returned to him. I carefully close the exam room door and return to Dr. C's office to wait with her for Mr. W's CT scan to arrive. The scan finally comes after several telephone visits, and together we make our way to Mr. W's exam room. Dr. C tells him that the scan has revealed a 6.5 mm diameter kidney stone that has lodged in his ureter. I internally writhe; I had a kidney stone once that was not nearly that large, and I remember the horrible pain it caused me. Because the stone is larger than 4.0 mm, Mr. We will not be able to pass the stone on his own. I notice Mr. W nod in his seat silently, wondering if he already knew if he had a kidney stone. The CT scan also reveals that the kidney is swelling. Dr. C explains that the stone has been blocking Mr. W's urine from reaching his bladder, saying that the pain comes from excess urine collecting in the kidney. To prevent further damage, Dr. C refers Mr. W to a local urologist to see by the end of the week. Mr. W calmly thanks her for her time. Dr. C leaves the room to ask the nurse to call the urologist, and we are on to see the next patient.

COVID AFFECTS MEMORY
THOMAS PATRICK (PRE-MATRIC JUNE 2023)

She was born as an only child to a Caucasian mother and an African American father. Her father was 47 at the time of her birth. At a young age, her father left her and her mother, going back to his other family. She knew a boy that she grew up with that she thought of as a sibling and referred to as her "brother" even though they shared no blood relation.

While in school her favorite subject was math. Her least favorite subject was reading as she did not enjoy it and saw it more as a chore. In college, she obtained an associate's degree in business. Later on, she became a CNA which she worked as for 21 years. During her adult years she often held 2-3 jobs. She even worked as a factory worker for some time. Recently, she worked as a store manager in retail. Her work often required her to work long hours throughout the week. This stressed her out and gave her really bad nightmares. She reports that she would often wake up screaming throughout the night. Covid had a long lasting impact on her.

In 2021, she contracted the COVID-19 virus. Even though her sickness only lasted around a week, she says the after-effects of the virus affected her memory. She often would forget how to get to work and get lost on the way there. Due to her memory issues and missing work, she watched as her work hours slowly dwindled. She went from working full time, to only working 1-2 days a week to none at all.

All of this, including her mother's passing, gave her extreme anxiety and depression. Her hope for her future is that she will "get better" by getting her anxiety and depression under control while also improving the quality of her sleep. This she hopes will lead to her living a normal life.

What brings her the most joy is fishing. She also enjoys playing with her dog which is a mix between a Jack Russell and pit bull. She describes her dog as "super energetic" who "bounces off the walls". Even though he weighs 45 lbs. he wants to be a lap dog. Even though she downplays the importance of feeling better she knows that feeling better will ultimately lead her to living a better life.

After interviewing her, it became apparent to me that she had a rough life. Growing up under a single parent can be challenging. I believe the impact of her mother's death took more of a toll on her than even she lets on. This is because her mother is the only person she's ever had to look up to. What gave me hope was the look on her face when she described fishing and her dog. I know she still has things that give her joy in this world and my hope is those things will help drive her out of this depression.

CHAPTER 5

Agency and Self-Confidence

ARE YOU A DOCTOR?
BILL CRUMP, MD

In my role as Associate Dean of the ULSOM rural regional Trover Campus in Madisonville, I have watched our student-directed free clinic transform since we began in 2004. This process accelerated when the COVID epidemic forced us to transition to entirely telemedicine visits. Although communicating via phone with our uninsured, low income patients was a challenge and some didn't have video capability, our students got quite comfortable with these virtual visits, staffed by me. We began cardiovascular screening at local food banks as our next step, and then most recently at the newly established Salvation Army homeless shelter. Until about a year ago, our town of 20,000 with a very sophisticated medical system lacked such a facility. The homeless in rural places are less concentrated so less visible, but we all knew they were there.

The story recounted below shows our most recent phase of providing impromptu portable clinic sessions. Even though the patient discussed had insurance and some family support, just being in a shelter provided obstacles. That same day, we saw another patient with no family support and no phone who had been off her blood pressure and diabetes medicines for almost a year. By working with our local health system to get lab done and choosing medications from the $4 list at a local pharmacy near a bus stop that accepts the shelter's vouchers, she is now being treated appropriately. But what is most important is the sense of pride and ownership that my students feel providing this service. Community Medicine concepts cannot be taught in a classroom, and the value of community engagement is learned best by personal experiences. I have watched this process develop in our students, and it provides meaning for all of us.

MICAH KAISER (MS 3 SEPTEMBER 2022)

"Are you a doctor? I've been having this stabbing pain in my belly for the past week and I've had ulcers in the past." This was how the patient greeted me as I entered the homeless shelter to do cardiovascular screening. She had seen my scrubs but not yet my badge and assumed I was a physician. Little did she know how distant I felt from being a physician as a third-year medical student. I told her that I was not but in my free-clinic role I could see her as a patient and maybe help. I made this bold statement knowing that a real physician would see her after me to verify that she received high-quality care and that I didn't miss anything.

For the past year, we had been doing cardiovascular screening in the shelter, measuring blood pressure, blood sugar, and total cholesterol. If any of these measurements were abnormal, we recommended the patient see their provider or see us in our student directed free clinic to address the issue. If any measurements were far beyond normal limits, we recommended they seek more immediate care. We had recommended that one woman go to the ED urgently who was later found to be having an MI. Unfortunately, there was a glaring gap in our strategy. It was almost impossible for the patients we screened in this homeless shelter to take return calls when they tried to make a medical appointment and we couldn't reach them to remind them of their appointment with us. Most had cell phones, but their minutes were very limited, didn't have text capability and most didn't use voice mail. They only answered numbers they recognized, not so different from us. So even though there was a low-cost city bus service that had a stop at the shelter, follow up visits weren't happening. So, we ultimately made the decision to hold patient visits in the shelter at the same time we did the screening to ensure that no patients got lost to follow-up.

The woman with the stabbing belly pain was the first patient encounter I had in our new system. As I began talking with her, I really began to understand the difficulties that underserved patient populations in chaotic social situations deal with on a regular basis. She stated that she hadn't seen a provider since she moved here from Ohio several months ago, but did see an APRN at a local urgent care occasionally. Her medical history in her words included previous strokes with some slow thinking afterwards, heart attacks, stomach ulcers, frequent UTIs, COPD, DM, and HTN. She was taking "way too many" medicines, but couldn't remember the names or dosages. She said her blood pressure typically ran about "70/30".

She reported diffuse right sided belly pain and flank pain that had been worsening for a week. She had nausea without vomiting and fatigue, dysuria, and dark-colored stools. On exam her BP was 113/65 and she had diffuse right sided abdominal tenderness that may have been a little worse in the right upper quadrant and positive CVA tenderness bilaterally. The tenderness though varied greatly with repeat exams a few seconds apart in severity and location.

Our initial concerns were for a UTI or cholelithiasis. She could not remember ever having an ultrasound examination of her abdomen. We told her our thoughts and she was agreeable with our plan. We ordered an abdominal ultrasound which later showed no abnormalities, CBC was normal, and urine showed more than 100,000 colonies of Klebsiella pneumoniae resistant only to Ampicillin. We called her and she recognized our number and answered. We suggested she see her APRN soon at the local urgent care or see us at our next visit to the shelter and called in trimethoprim/sulfa (Bactrim) BID for 7 days.

She was one of earliest patients in our new system, but she really highlights its success. Currently, many physicians are not available for patient appointments until weeks ahead. Urgent care provides little continuity and these are overwhelmed with each new Covid wave. The individuals in the shelter simply can't navigate all the obstacles. So, the ability to offer "on the spot" visits to these patients who are already underserved is very valuable. What we provide may be the best—and the only—opportunity for them to receive timely medical care. As a medical student, the value to my education of providing this service is the ability to take responsibility for a patient who would not receive care otherwise. It is significantly more responsibility and ownership over patient care than I usually experience, and with that, it creates a learning experience like no other. This level of patient ownership reminds me of why I wanted to be a physician in the first place: to help those who are in need.

WHEN IT CLICKED
HANNAH MARSHALL (MS 3 AUGUST 2023)

Medicine is centered around a "see one, do one, teach one" model, and I have always seemed to adapt reluctantly. Each progressive year you become more and more comfortable with being pushed far beyond your comfort zone and you get less petrified of doing things you thought you may never do. A stark example: being the primary care provider for a patient in the beginning of your third year of medical school. First rotation. First real clinical experience. Sole, primary provider, decision maker, imposter-but-real life doctor.

As a part of our rural curriculum, we are given the experience to provide cardiovascular screening to members of the community. We are sent out to the places that have the most need and give healthcare access to those who have barriers to traditional healthcare, often no fault of their own. In turn, patients who need a primary care physician are assigned a third-year medical student that acts as the healthcare provider with intent to bridge the patient to establishing a long-term relationship with a physician.

My first screening was on a Saturday at a local food bank. I was so excited at the potential thought of picking up my own patient and getting out of the books and into the community. I was fresh out of step one, with limited clinical experience, and antsy to get involved. All the excitement wore off into absolute terror when the stranger in front of me, who had a blood pressure higher than I had ever seen, was signing a paper stating they were allowing me to access their medical records and take over their care. Even with my faculty supervisor just a few feet away involved with another patient, I felt the weight of this responsibility.

It shocked me how much this person I had never met before trusted me. He clung onto every word I said, completely amenable to any and every suggestion I had made regarding lab work and medication. I barely knew what came in a CBC or a BMP, but when I explained the importance of checking his baseline creatinine before starting an ACE-I or an ARB he thanked me for being thorough and knowledgeable. It felt like a false sense of hope, someone looking to me for answers when I felt I was just the knock-off version of a "real doctor".

I left realizing the power this position holds. The true "umph" that even the title of Student Doctor can carry. It feels equally rewarding and sickening. On one hand I am validated that years of hard work will mean something but terrified at the magnitude of that something.

A mentor, much greyer than myself, would always tell us to "get on the same side of the room as the patient" both physically and metaphorically. I used to make light and make jokes of such "Crump-isms", but now it clicked. Our job now is to take the power we've spent the last greater half of our lives working to feel and transferring that power to be thoroughly used up and passed on to your community, passing the metaphorical baton and physically getting on the same side of the room.

EXTENDING MEDICAL STUDENT ACCESS TO PATIENTS
MARISSA STEWART (MS 3 MARCH 2009)

"I am only one, but still I am one. I cannot do everything, but still I can do something; and because I cannot do everything, I will not refuse to do the something that I can do." Wow! What an amazing and inspiring thought by Edmund Everett Hale. As I began to reflect on the time that I had completed by serving our community in the community clinic, I thought I have in some small way contributed my talents to our society.

The Community Clinic is a medical facility which offers free healthcare to the employed, uninsured, who could not otherwise afford healthcare on their own. The clinic finds itself serving a population who desperately want and need the care that we provide. As third- and fourth-year medical students we are asked to volunteer in the clinic if we so desire. I chose to give of my time by volunteering and serving this population of people. As a medical student sometimes you feel as though you play such a small part in healthcare. In a typical healthcare setting the medical student is very limited to what they can do, such as history and physicals, formulating a differential diagnosis, and devising a plan. Ultimately, though, the clinical decision making is left up to the attending physician. In the free clinic, however, the medical student feels as though they have control of the patient's care and are able to make some clinical decisions with guidance from an attending physician. I found this very fulfilling in that I was caring for patients, but on a completely different level I was serving the underprivileged and those who are less fortunate than me.

The time that I served in free clinic was very rewarding and eye-opening because I learned to have an open mind and that things are not always black and white. It is very easy in the medical field to become jaded, but working in the clinic and becoming personally connected with my patients allowed me to step back and remind myself why I had gotten into medicine to begin with. I wanted to serve and give back to my community, and what better way than to serve the less privileged. So I have given something back as small or as minor as I think it may be and with as little as I have to offer, it matters. It matters to my patients, it matters to the clinic, it matters to our community, it matters to our society, but most of all it matters to me. Because in serving others, I have grown and enriched myself and ultimately have and will become a better person and physician for it.

HAKUNA MATATA
ROHIT NAIR (MS 3 SEPTEMBER 2020)

July 7, 2018 will forever go down as the first day I truly felt like a medical professional. It was the sixth of our eight clinic days on the University of Louisville School of Medicine service learning trip to the beautiful African nation of Tanzania, in partnership with the Foxes NGO and the Mufindi Children's Orphanage. Being on this trip was how I wanted to spend the summer between my first and second years of medical school, but I had no idea about how impactful the memories shared among me and 14 classmates on the trip would be. As a group, we treated over 1000 patients living in remote villages in the mountainous Iringa district – who often only receive healthcare services when brigades set up travelling clinics in their village once a year. Over 35% of the population in this region is HIV positive. In addition, we had the opportunity to see other conditions we rarely see back home. My fellow classmates and I all honed in on skills learned during our first year of medical school, including the physical exam and history taking. We also experienced countless firsts – our first time doing intramuscular injections, our first pelvic/rectal exams, our first time debriding wounds, our first time helping out in a pharmacy, our first time taking histories on real patients, and our first time presenting patients to an outstanding group of humanitarian attendings. With this background, I will share one particular encounter which ties together so many of the elements that made my first trip to Africa a life event that solidified my decision to be a physician.

On July 7th, I was on travel clinic duty in the village of Loudilo, which is an hour drive from our home base at the Mufindi Children's Orphanage. When we set up in these villages, we would create makeshift clinics in community centers which were often mudbrick structures without any electricity or running water. I spent the morning how I had spent most of the preceding days, seeing patients in a dark room with the aid of Swahili interpreters. After lunch, it was my turn to be on wound care duty and I let one of my classmates take over the patient room. However, most of the people who needed wound care came in the morning, so there was not much action at the wound care station. At Loudilo, there were numerous patients waiting outside the clinic for their turn to be seen after being checked in. Since I was not busy, I decided I would try to be helpful. Luckily, Mr. K, one of the directors of the Mufindi Children's Orphanage, happened to also be standing around near me. I did not have an interpreter assigned to me at the time, and Mr. K knows some Swahili - so we decided we would start taking histories of the patients waiting outside in an effort to accommodate as many patients who showed up that day as we could.

The very first patient we talked to was a 27-year-old woman who complained of getting dizzy when she stood up. Even with my amateur history-taking skills, I knew to ask if she was pregnant as part of my line of questioning. This was awkward, because the people in this culture tend to be very bashful, and there were many other people within earshot as we took this history on a bench outside the clinic building. Due to this, Geoff said he translated this question in a very euphemistic way, but she denied being pregnant. I checked her blood pressure and it was normal.

We knew we had pregnancy test strips in the pharmacy, so we decided to check this despite her insistence that she was not pregnant. At this point, Mr. K had to leave, so it was just me and the patient with a large language barrier between us – as all the interpreters were busy helping out my classmates in rooms. With mainly hand signals, I instructed the patient to go to the nearby outhouse and urinate in a cup. I grabbed a pregnancy test strip and waited outside the outhouse for the patient to finish while I studied the label for what would constitute a positive result. She came back with the urine, I put the test strip in following the instructions, and sure enough 2 lines appeared on the strip indicating a positive test.

So there I was, alone with this woman holding a cup of her own urine by an outhouse, unsure if I read the test correctly - with no way of telling her this life-changing news. I immediately signaled for the patient to wait there since I wanted to maintain as much of her privacy as possible while I ran over to Dr. E, a pediatrician who confirmed that the test was indeed positive. At this point, I borrowed my colleague's interpreter, brought him back to where the patient was, and mentally prepared myself to deliver the most important thing I had ever told anyone at this point in my young medical career. When the Swahili words for "the test was positive, it looks like you are pregnant" came out of the interpreter's mouth, the patient's jaw dropped – she looked absolutely shocked and then said something. The interpreter turned to me and said "she cannot believe it" with a dead-pan face. For a moment I thought "oh no, what if that is not what she wanted to hear, what do I say next?" But right as I processed that thought, the patient's face lit up with excitement, she did a celebratory jump, and she had the biggest smile I have ever seen as she proceeded to hug me. I wanted to share this pure moment of human emotion with her in her language, so naturally the first thing that came to my mind to exclaim was "hakuna matata!" It means "no worries, for the rest of your days" – which you probably know from The Lion King. Turns out, she and her husband had been trying to have another child for the past 2 years and she thanked me for "giving her the best news she has ever heard." We gave her some pre-natal vitamins and sent her on her merry way, while Dr. S (our lead faculty advisor) explained to me how pregnancy can cause orthostatic hypotension.

In the time since our service learning trip to Tanzania, we have been immersed in the intense middle years of medical school. It can sometimes be tedious to study for days at a time, but any time I find myself with these thoughts, I think of how happy that one lady in Africa was when I told her she was pregnant, and I feel proud that we were resourceful enough to be able to touch so many lives in those eight days. It also confirmed that I made the right choice with how I want to spend the rest of my life. In how many other fields can you tell such an interesting story from such a remote place in the world with such a happy ending? This was just a story about a first, and I know I will one day have to break bad news too. But I am so thankful to be in a field where I can travel anywhere in the world and provide value to fellow humans, and to that I can say – hakuna matata.

PALLIATIVE CARE FOR THE PATIENT WITH CHRONIC PAIN
KATHRIENA GREENWELL (MS 3 NOVEMBER 2015)

Mr. C is a forty-five-year-old man who has skin cancer that has spread to lymph nodes in his neck. He has undergone surgery to remove the skin cancer and has also been undergoing radiation therapy of his neck for the past three months. Due to the effect of radiation, Mr. C has severe chronic pain in the skin of his neck as well as in his throat. The main focus of his palliative care is control of his pain. He has been taking pain medications to try to minimize his pain to allow him to get through his daily functions as best as possible. However, his pain is somewhat uncontrolled. Due to the pain he experiences with swallowing, he has lost much of his appetite and has lost over twenty-five pounds unintentionally in the last three months. Fortunately, Mr. C has a lot of social support at home with his family who always comes to his office visits with him. However, when I inquired about the goals of his care with him and his family, they seemed to be somewhat unsure. When speaking with his primary care physician, she revealed that there is a lot of miscommunication between care providers for this patient.

The care of Mr. C and his family could be improved in several ways. The communication between care providers should be enhanced so that all parties have a better understanding of the patients' goals as well as the goals of the care providers for Mr. C. These goals should be discussed with Mr. C and his family so that they have a thorough understanding and do not have misconceptions about what his future holds. Additionally, Mr. C's pain is uncontrolled to the point that it is affecting his activities of daily living and causing him to lose weight. This should also be addressed through changing medicines, increasing dosages, or alternative pain management.

This experience affected me personally because it altered both my attitude toward pain management and my perception of palliative care. In regards to pain management, I typically think of patients who want to abuse the system and abuse pain medications. However, this patient reminded me of the importance of pain control for those patients with chronic pain so that they can live a life as close to normal for them as possible. Furthermore, I did not realize all of the different aspects of care that exist within palliative care or that palliative care was not only for those that are dying imminently. Also, I learned that an important aspect of palliation is to discuss with the patient what he or she wants from his or her healthcare. In my future practice, I will be sure to address what goals patients have for themselves and their care so that I may provide care that is in line with their desires.

HEALING GOES BOTH WAYS: CRYING WITH LISA
JOSHUA FUQUA (MS 3 DECEMBER 2019)

As I walked into Lisa's room on a Thursday morning, I knew what to expect. I'd glanced through her chart: Suicidal Ideation. She had come into the ED the day before, brought by a concerned friend, for threatening suicide. This was my second week on inpatient psych but I'd already begun to form differentials and treatment plans for the H&Ps I wrote every morning. I'd started mentally rolling through the short list of antidepressants I knew and that the patient hadn't already tried. The next 45 minutes was filled with a chain of events that would make the most emotionally numb trauma surgeon tear up. She'd had a rough year.

A year ago, she had a pap smear and it came back CIN III. She had a colposcopy – it was painful. She then went through chemotherapy and intravaginal radiation – it was also painful. She had a hysterectomy and, sure enough, the recovery was painful. She recounted her darkest moments of vomiting into the toilet bowl while trying to keep the blood running down her legs from staining her white bathroom tile. This happened more times than she could easily recount. Her family was supportive; they cared and called often. However, they never came to treatments or stayed with her afterward while she bled and vomited. After 6 months, her boyfriend couldn't handle watching it anymore. He left her, only to come back to her after feeling guilty about leaving a sick woman in chemotherapy to fend for herself. Her work friends and coworkers were understanding; they sent cards and flowers, and she got a year of paid leave. Each card mentioned that they couldn't wait to see her back at work.

After a year of treatments, her oncologist proclaimed her in remission and "cured." When she returned to work 6 days before her current admission, everyone welcomed her back and were so excited she was better. Many mentions of "wow, cancer is so hard, my uncle died from cancer", "my mother died to endometrial cancer it's incredible you're still here", and "you must be so happy to have beaten cancer, how's it feel to be back to normal?". She didn't feel normal.

Her uterus was gone and vaginal sclerosis racked her pelvis. Her colon was often impacted and her bladder had become incontinent. She had numerous peritoneal adhesions that caused belly pain tormented her daily. Her mind was still foggy and her memory suffered. Her family did her grocery shopping, and took her to appointments. Her boyfriend was with her "out of pity", she thought. Her coworkers saw her as "a walking cancer doll". She felt alone, abandoned, and like a "freak" living in the shell of who she used to be. She could only handle 4 hours at work before the pain forced her home, and it was the final straw. By the time I saw her six days later, she was on her last legs. I cried with her, and told her she was at the right place, but I had no clue what to do for her. This wasn't fixable with medication.

I left her room feeling the crushing weight of deep depression that comes from a life that doesn't stop swinging when you're down. A few hours later in a side room with my attending, she recounted her story. My attending nodded his head slowly with each major story point, making affirmative noises. When she was done, she asked to be released so she could go back to her life. She believed there was nothing we could do to help. My attending spent the next 30 minutes questioning why she felt so hopeless. As he inquired with more and more pointed intent, Lisa began to question her view of her circumstances and her own insecurities and fears. She began to realize she felt so useless and hopeless because she was measuring herself by other's expectations of her. She was locked into a lifestyle she hated, but felt she had no say over and no option out of. She had allowed, directly or indirectly, her life to be run by other people and their expectations of her: how she should feel, when to go back to work, when to leave the house, what to eat, what to buy, and the list goes on. She could only blame those around her, "they make me feel... they told me... they expected me...". She had lost sight of her own life amidst incredibly unfortunate circumstances, and it seemed to her that it had destroyed her. She so desperately wanted to go back to the way things were before her life hit a downward spiral, but that simply didn't seem possible. Afterward, I stopped by her room and shared my own past of depression and eventual recovery. I broke into tears with her again, but this time both of us shed tears of hope; hope that if someone else could do it, she could too.

Over the following three days the psychiatric team taught her how to deal with her situation. There was no changing things; you can't turn back the clock, no matter how magical medicine may seem. What we could do was teach her how to deal with her circumstances. We started with how she looked at her own situation, and then changing whose standards she was measuring herself against. Then, we worked confidence and self-image exercises into her daily routine to improve her self-confidence and self-worth. We had a family conference where she took the initiative in asking her family for changes - let her make more decisions with her life so she felt less like an animal in a zoo. Lastly, we arranged for further time off work until she was more physically able. We hadn't taken away the pain or fear of her situation, but we had given her tools to fight back.

Her time on the psych floor reminded me greatly of my own fight with depression a few years ago, as well as my struggle as a student in the medical system and in medical education. As I toiled as a pre-med, my depression was at its worst. Feelings of sadness or worry were not what overwhelmed me- it was feelings of hopelessness that I had no other options in life. At the time, I hated my work, I rarely saw my friends, I was frustrated with my family, I resented my previous degree, and I saw no end in sight. I felt really and truly hopeless. It wasn't until I started exercising and meditating as a last desperate whim that I began to crawl out of that hole. I wasn't able to change my circumstance, not quickly at least, but I could change how I handled it. I was able to adjust and put power back into my own hands. In doing so, I could approach the impossible and begin reversing the situation in time. I was able to adapt how I reacted to my world in the short term, and subsequently change its shape around me in the long term.

Now, as a third-year medical student I've begun to recognize the signs I saw in Lisa and myself in my colleagues ranging from first year students to grizzled attendings. The feeling of being trapped within your circumstances, of your own making or someone else's, leads to a repetitive cycle of helplessness. We have to see X number of patients per day, we have to write good notes, we have to appeal to patients, colleagues, and God-forsaken insurance companies. Doctors are expected to harbor the responsibilities of three people at a time between conferences, family, research, and administration. Meanwhile we are expected to feel "blessed" for this.

When I applied for medical school, no one mentioned 60-hour work weeks being normal. No one mentioned the mind-numbing fear that is step exams and boards studying, the irate university attendings who lost their humanity long, long ago, and the patients who will berate you with profanity and insensitivity. Medical students, residents, and physicians are often trapped in a laundry list of obligation, expectation, and niceties. As Lisa waved goodbye on the day of her release, I waved back realizing what we'd felt was the same source of burnout and frustration doctors are facing and will continue to face. We can't change our circumstances, not immediately. We assuredly need change for mental health in medicine; I don't think there's a person on Earth who would argue otherwise. However, the wheels of change are slow and rusty, and until then we are left with only what we can control. Take a walk every day, keep a thought log, see a therapist, let yourself actually feel with patients. Do something, anything, to stay a human being. The world of medicine will rip your humanity from you if you give it the chance; it's you who has to hold onto it. Some days it takes crying with Lisa to remember that.

SKATING ON THIN ICE
SARAH FISHER (MS 3 OCTOBER 2014)

Since starting as a third-year medical student, I have been immersed in the care of many patients. I have learned about the aspects of heart failure exacerbations, managing diabetes, when to start a statin, and reading chest x-rays. While all of these are important and necessary for my medical training, there is still one component that can't be learned through lectures and observation: humanism. It is through patient interaction that we, as medical students, learn about the art of medicine and its humanistic nature. My patients are as much my teachers as my attending physicians, and maybe even a little more in many ways.

During my morning rounds on a cold January morning, I walked into one of my patient's rooms and greeted by the smiles of my patient and his family. I asked about his shortness of breath, listened to his wife's concerns, and carefully examined my patient. I answered his questions the best I could, reassuring that I would relay any concerns to his physician, and as I excused myself promising to check on him later, my patient said to me, "Thank you very much. I sure do appreciate you." I was floored. Don't get me wrong, people say thank you all of the time; it is sometimes more out of habit rather than sincerity. However, I have never been told that I was appreciated, and that was humbling. Why would a patient be appreciative of me, a student? I was then reminded that if a patient can appreciate me, a learner, then I need be even more grateful for the people who are playing a role in my education: my attendings who are encouragers, the nurses who help me with beeping alarms and explain ventilator stats, and the custodians who graciously keep our hospital clean. My patient taught me the truth from this Serbian proverb: "Be humble, for you are made of earth."

The other half of that proverb is, "Be noble, for you are made of stars." My patients have encouraged me to see my own potential. Going into third year is very similar to trying to skate in the same ice rink as Olympic figure skaters – intimidating, terrifying, and mostly humiliating. You spend most of your time hugging the wall and attempting to skate, while your attendings pass by you doing beautiful jumps. One of the ways to join those skating is having the crowd cheer you on, encouraging you, and even believing in you when you can't fathom the thought of continuing on. My patients have been the cheering fans I've needed to build confidence in myself. Whether it was correctly diagnosing a diastasis recti rather than a hernia, or hearing the words, "You're going to be a great doctor someday," my patients have subtly cheered me along, encouraging me to slowly let go of the wall and skate on my own. It will take time until I can do all of the intricate jumps like my attendings; until then, I will continue to practice learning to skate without letting my self-doubt keep me attached to the wall.

NOT THE TEXTBOOK VERSION OF SCHIZOPHRENIA JESSICA ISON (MS 3 OCTOBER 2014)

I had another set of feelings when I saw a schizophrenic patient at the far end of her treatment. I was seeing a middle-aged woman who came to the office for a routine visit. She was currently being treated with antipsychotics to manage her schizophrenia and did not report any particular problems. She was living in a group home, which she came to after a psychotic episode that resulted in hospitalization in a mental hospital several years ago. When asked about her goals and plans for the future she indicated that she wanted to reach the point where she could move and care for her younger sister. She also wanted to begin to work again.

This office visit was routine and relatively uneventful from a medical standpoint. She was continued on her current medications and encouraged to pursue finding a job at which she could invest some of her time. What makes this encounter especially meaningful to me, though, is that it gave me a vivid picture of at least a piece of the life of someone living with schizophrenia. She wasn't the picture of an acute episode of schizophrenia that you read about in textbooks or try to remember so that you can recognize it on the exam. She was a person, with a history, who loved her sister and desired to care for her despite what she was experiencing herself, and who was looking to create a future for herself regardless of her current situation. At the same time, though, it saddened me to see the toll that her illness and its treatment had taken on her. It was quickly apparent upon meeting her that although she was faithfully taking her medications and not acutely psychotic by any stretch of the imagination, she wasn't anywhere near what I imagine her baseline was before her first psychotic episode. As much as I wanted her to be able to return to some kind of normal, I couldn't ignore how difficult a process it would be for her to be able to find a job, transition to living on her own, and make her way back to her sister. My encounter with this patient underscored the fact that a chronic mental illness seems to be able to reach areas of a person's life that other diseases cannot. Her physical body remained intact, but the very essence of who she was and the life she hoped for had been affected in a way I had not previously observed in a patient.

This encounter also left me feeling more than a little helpless. All of the correct treatments for schizophrenia were being employed, yet she wasn't "cured." This is an uncomfortable realization because when you study to become a doctor you believe that if you just learn enough information and treatment plans you'll be able to "fix" a patient. Admittedly, her life was improved by the treatment she was receiving. But this encounter reminded me that sometimes there is only so much that medication can do.

The knowledge and insight I gained from this experience will have an effect on my future practice of medicine. I will strive not to allow the feeling of helplessness from not being able to "cure" some patients to cause me to shy away from giving them the best care I possibly can. I will acknowledge where medications fall short and seek to be compassionate and explore ways in which I can partner with my patients to set goals and help them reach those goals. Also, I will search for other avenues through which they can be helped. For example, during this clerkship I discovered an Adult Day Therapeutic Rehabilitation Program that helps patients with chronic mental illnesses by placing them in a community of people with similar issues in order to combat the isolation that they often face.

I will also seek to continue to reflect on the "routine" patient encounters that can be all too easily overlooked during a busy day. I will remind myself once again to stop and think of each patient in the context of who they've been, who they are, and who they want to be- not simply in terms of what medications they should be prescribed and what tests should be performed."

KNOWLEDGE
IAN LEATHERMAN (CRS JULY 2021)

It's important to know what you know.

You must make decisions that can impact the course of people's lives.

You shouldn't make any of those decisions based on knowledge you don't have.

So, you must know when you don't know.

There is always someone who knows more.

So, if you don't know, let them make the decision.

LAW AND MEDICINE
CIERRA WOODCOCK (CRS JULY 2020)

Mr. A is a 73-year-old man that grew up in Western Ky. Upon first meeting with Mr. A, it was very clear to see that he was not a regular old man. He possessed an intelligence not seen often in small towns in Kentucky and had quite the sense of humor. When asked why he was at the doctor that particular day, he stated with a big grin "I have no real reason for being here. I was summoned by the doc, so I came."

Mr. A spent his younger years getting his undergraduate degree at Murray State University. While there, he mentioned he joined the ROTC program to avoid going to Vietnam. However, he said that he learned a lot of useful things in the program that helped him later on in life with his future career. After completing his degree at Murray State, he then went on to become a lawyer, He talked about all the cases he had to work with doctors over the years and advised me that in my future endeavors "if a lawyer asks for something, do yourself a favor and just give it to them. It will make your life easier." Before my time ended with Mr. A, he gave a final piece of advice to think about in the future. He said, "I'm sure you don't want to be a doctor for the money, but in the end, you've got to make a living and take care of yourself. So, when choosing a profession, pick one that pays well for all the hard work you put into it."

Although Mr. A was an interesting man with a great story to tell and good advice to give, he had a particular quality that I was not too fond of. While discussing his career and my future career, he mentioned that it would be much more difficult for me to be a good doctor compared to my male counter parts in the field. He also included that it was highly unlikely that I would actually make it to be a doctor, where my male counter parts would make it much more easily. When I asked him why, he said because as a woman, it was my job to birth and care for children. If I had children, it would be difficult for me to be a good mother and a good doctor. It would also be harder for me to become a doctor because my male counterparts weren't running on a "natural clock," so it would be harder for me to become a mother and become a doctor. This frustrated me because I am a 20-year-old female with all the time in the world and nothing on her mind but achieving her goals in life. I could not believe people would still say things like that. This is where I learned my biggest lesson that would follow me throughout my future career. I learned that even when patients say things that are unkind, you just have to take it with a grain of salt and not allow it to affect how you treat that patient. You have to care about and respect your patients, even with they do not. After all, you don't become a doctor to help yourself; you do it to help them.

CHAPTER 6

Empathy Grows in End of Life Care

LOOKING BEYOND THE PHYSICAL BODY
KRISTIN WICKHAM (MS 3 JULY 2015)

The patient was an elderly gentleman with a long history of smoking that was diagnosed with end stage lung disease, COPD. The doctors approximated that he only had six months or less to live because of the advanced stage of his disease. He has been under the care of hospice for almost one year now, and is slowly declining in function. He especially struggles with feeling like he is unable to adequately breathe and get oxygen into his lungs. The patient entered hospice to be kept comfortable and have his pain controlled during his final days.

The predominant needs of this patient include breathing assistance/support, pain management, safety with transferring between his bed and chair, and coping with end of life issues. A team of people within the hospice system is currently meeting these needs very well. The nurse offers medication instructions and helps with safety issues, for example getting the right equipment into the home to help the patient stay safe. The nurse also communicates with the doctor to make sure that the right medications and the right doses of those medications are being prescribed to meet the patient's needs. The social worker comes to the home and assesses the patient's living situation and their support system to determine what kind of extra support that the patient or family needs. The chaplain comes to the home to discuss readiness for the end of life with the patient. He or she also provides extra spiritual and emotional support to the patient and family. The goals of this patient's care are to keep the patient living comfortably and with the best quality of life possible until the progression of his disease naturally allows him to pass, and I believe that these goals are being met.

After visiting the patient's home, there are a couple of ways that I believe that the patient's care could be enhanced. The room where the patient spends all of his time is very cluttered with furniture and other items that may provide obstacles in the patient safely transferring between bed and chair. These items may not be necessary for the patient to feel comfortable, and may be able to be moved to a different room in the house to promote safety. Also, the patient has started to develop some dependent edema and skin changes on the right lower leg. Treating this edema and making the patient more comfortable may enhance his care. He may benefit from keeping his legs elevated while sitting in his chair or from some skin ointment.

The hospice team does a great job communicating with one another. Not only do they communicate throughout the week, but they also have meetings every two weeks with the whole team where they review the care plans for each patient. The nurse, then the social worker, then the chaplain all report on their weekly visits with the patient, and then the team discusses the patient's anticipated needs. Other team members present at these meetings include the hospice director, a physician and the coordinator for volunteers. By reviewing each patient's care plan and assessing their needs every two weeks, this interdisciplinary setting supports quality care for the patient's and their families.

Going to the home visit to meet this patient was a good experience for me. It really allowed me to see the patient's environment, so that I could better understand his situation. The room in which he was spending his last days was average size, tidy, and had lots of things in it. As I looked around, I saw that pictures of his family surrounded him. These pictures served as a reminder that he is somebody's husband, somebody's dad and somebody's grandfather. The experience reminded me of the importance of looking beyond the physical body in front of me, and to consider a patient's surroundings and environment when attempting to understand them as a whole person. Professionally, this experience taught me the importance of connecting with your patients on more than just a medical level. It is important for the physician to discuss the physical needs of the patient of course, but many times it is also necessary for the physician to venture past their traditional role and help to take care of the emotional, spiritual or practical needs that the patient may have. Seeing this particular doctor/patient relationship on the home visit had nothing but a positive impact on me. It showed me how important a personal relationship with patients can be, in addition to the typical medical relationship. The way the doctor spoke with the patient displayed his true concern for this patient that he had been seeing every few months for almost a year. The way the patient communicated showed that he trusted the doctor. This type of relationship is the goal for optimal patient care, not only palliative, but in all forms of practice.

Before the palliative rotation, I assumed that palliative care was equal to end of life care. While that is a part of palliative care, I have learned that the title encompasses much more. Palliative care includes meeting all aspects of the needs of patients, including physical, emotional, social and spiritual needs. These can be in patients needing care temporarily, for chronic illnesses or for end of life care. I have learned that palliative care is really a team effort. There is no part that is more important than the rest; each person on the team just meets a different need so that the totalities of the patient's needs are met. Meeting a wide range of needs for a patient allows for the best outcome for the patient's overall health.

CARE THAT DOESN'T END IN A CURE
TALITHA JONES (MS 4 MARCH 2022)

As a medical student, there is a day we all dread, the day one of our patients' lives ends. For some, this comes early in their career, others a bit later. Sometimes we are notified simply by seeing the patient's name removed from our patient list the next day, other times, end-of-life is a journey we take with the patient. One journey I took was with a patient receiving palliative care due to pancreatic cancer. The man was relatively young, only 60 years old, married, and had kids about my age and grandchildren. I met this patient on my first day of my third-year internal medicine rotation, but this experience will always stay with me. He was extremely sick and had been suffering for several months. In the last few weeks, his vitals had taken a turn for the worst, and the end was near. I saw first-hand as we began shifting our patient care goals from an emphasis on bettering outcomes and chasing lab values to providing comfort for the patient and his family. At first, our conversations had a very medical tone. We went over the status of each of his failing systems. We explained how we were managing each, but, in the end, we backed off this kind of discussion and instead transitioned to pain control and discussing realistic plans with the family and supporting them during this trying time.

Each day, our team tried to view this situation not as if there was nothing left we could do but instead, how can we could best support this transition. We spoke to the family often and learned the patient and his family were devout Christians. One service we provided was an opportunity to speak with the Chaplin daily. This was a huge comfort to the family and made them feel supported spiritually in a way we, as healthcare providers, couldn't. Another hurdle we had to address was that the hospital's current rules only allowed one family member in the ICU. This was extremely difficult on the patient's grown children, who wanted to be with their father in his last days. They also desperately wanted their young children to see their Papaw one last time. As a team, we decided to keep them updated by calling them daily when we came by to see the patient and allowing his wife to FaceTime the other family members while we were there. On what we believed to be the final day, we were also able to enable the family to use an iPad and FaceTime the family for goodbyes. The nurses coordinated this, and each gave special attention and care to this family. We, as staff, were in the room with the wife, so she knew she was not alone physically as well. Lastly, we allowed the patient's wife to decorate the patient's room with family pictures and brought blankets from home so the room would feel homier. Overall, I felt the entire care team, the nurses, physicians, medical students, social workers, and Chaplin all played their roles well to help facilitate this challenging care.

If I were to change anything about this patient's care, I wish we would have been able to address some of the family's end-of-life discussions sooner so that the patient could have been more coherent. Though the prognosis was never good, the family held off as long as they could to discuss what his final days would look like despite ample counseling. I wonder if we had been more direct with the family about how the pressure of many decisions can weigh heavily during the final days and how the Covid regulations were not changing, may have better prepared them. Though difficult to think about early on, it could eliminate stress later when everyone is more fragile. This is also a challenge because, as physicians, it is impossible to know precisely when a patient might take a turn for the worst. Despite this, the team did an excellent job of keeping the care patient-oriented and always reminding everyone that we want to do what is in the patient's best interest and would be what he would have wanted. This helped the family navigate difficult decisions. I was happy to see the care team act as guardrails in those conversations and even mediators between family members.

We were fortunate to have an incredible interdisciplinary team. The Chaplin, nurses and social workers were all involved and communicated efficiently and gracefully. They had each other's phone numbers and knew to respond quickly as this situation could need immediate action. One strength I saw was that the staff continued care beyond the patient's life by setting the wife up with a support group and following up with the family.

This experience was my first as a member of an in end-of-life care team. I remember his final days were filled with so much discussion and emotion, but in the end, it is all very quiet and peaceful. I will never forget how anticlimactic I found death to be. I was touched by how every member of the team showed their humanism and went above and beyond their duty to support and care for this family, even if it meant a big wig physician helping tape up posters with pictures of the grandkids because he knew how important it was to the family. This is the kind of provider I want to be. I don't want to stop at simply providing medical care but want to treat my patients and their families holistically, caring for them mentally and spiritually. I want to always connect with my human side that reminds me no matter how many times I have seen death that this is still so hard for the family and go out of my way to provide comfort where I can. I initially thought palliative care was an easy form of medicine because I didn't know what could be done medically. However, I learned that nothing in end of life care is easy. Though the focus may shift from physical healing, to other forms of care such as spiritual, social, and mental support they are still very challenging and necessary.

GARDENING DURING HOSPICE
REBECCA RAJ (MS 4 AUGUST 2018)

"Mr. Joe" is a 72 year old African American gentleman diagnosed with terminal prostate cancer. He carried the diagnosis for several years but in a recent turn of events, he experienced a sudden decline that could no longer be therapeutically managed with chemo-radiation. Consequently, his oncologist referred him to hospice care. Since the new goal of radiation is simply for symptomatic care and his prognosis is limited to less than 6 months, it is appropriate to be referred to palliative care services. Mr. Joe has come to terms with his illness and demonstrates eagerness to maintain his quality of life for as long as he is able.

He lives at home with his wife and receives frequent visits from his children and grandchildren who live in surrounding counties. On days that his children visit, he finds himself content with the way things are. However, on days when they are unable to visit and his wife must run errands or take care of her sick mother, the burden of his terminal illness weighs heavily on him. For this reason, the spiritual counselor meets with him weekly to encourage and offer strategies to counteract downward spiral thinking. The counselor also explores ideas of legacy and reflection on Mr. Joe's life experiences which help remind him of truths to hold onto and give him peace. Since he was referred to palliative services, Mr. Joe has expressed an improvement in how he is able to manage the days that he feels alone and hopeless. There is no clear, objective manner in which to evaluate this improvement, but the counselor has noted a brighter and more hopeful attitude in Mr. Joe when discussing the harder days than when he first visited Mr. Joe.

Due to his decline, walking without assistance has become too difficult to manage, so he remains in a bed or wheelchair most of the day. The volunteer who helps him with daily tasks a few times a week realized that working in the garden would truly lift Mr. Joe's spirits. To that end, she worked with a social worker to get insurance coverage for a 4 wheel drive medical scooter that can be used outdoors. Since introducing this intervention, Mr. Joe has grown significantly more cheerful in disposition as he is able to spend time in his garden.

This experience has taught me to look beyond a patient's medical illness. While this is an intuitive lesson, I feel the message is easily forgotten during training years when the focus is shifted strictly to disease management. The overarching theme of healing holistically somehow gets lost in translation. The joy Mr. Joe received from returning to his garden reminded me that much of healing begins in the mind such that when healing of the body is not possible, our work as physicians does not have to be over. Seeing the interdisciplinary team come together to improve Mr. Joe's quality of life empowers me to seek opportunities to act similarly in my role as a medical student and in future as a resident physician. Spending time with the interdisciplinary team will make me more likely to encourage patients to think positively of the benefits of palliative care services because they are truly many.

SUPPORT FOUND IN PALLIATIVE CARE
DEVIN CLARK (MS 3 OCTOBER 2021)

Ms. Jane, a 60-year-old woman I had the pleasure of working with towards the end of my third year, was a retired schoolteacher recently diagnosed with metastatic pancreatic cancer. She first noticed her symptoms while performing chores around the house in spring of 2021. She remembers being severely fatigued with the simplest of errands and recalls frequent bouts of stomach pain. Eventually, her symptoms resulted in a trip to the local urgent care. Jane underwent a CT scan of her abdomen and was instructed to follow up with a GI specialist. There, the diagnosis was revealed to her and the prognosis discussed.

Jane was initially devastated. She was in total disbelief and didn't understand how this could happen to her (a healthy 60-year-old who exercised daily and had a healthy diet). The only mark against her was the nasty habit of smoking cigarettes she had picked up as a teenager. Luckily, the patient had overwhelming support from her husband and two girls. She was also cheered on by friends, neighbors, and former coworkers. Jean began chemotherapy 1-2 weeks after her initial diagnosis. She lost her hair, her energy, and struggled to complete her daily routines. Her mood began to change which was first noticed by her husband. Jane had become more tearful, anxious and pessimistic about her future. These observations were eventually brought it up to her oncologist, who encouraged a referral to palliative care to help Jane manage some of her through treatment not offered by their office. Jane agreed.

At Jane's first palliative care meeting, she was stunned by the format of the appointment. Jane entered the conference room where her family, along with the physician, the nurse, the social worker and the chaplain were seated. Jane was positioned at the head of the conference table. The meeting began with a brief overview of palliative care, led by Amy, one of the social workers. It was explained to Jane that the goal of palliative care was to ease her symptoms and help relieve physical and emotional burden. In addition, palliative care was there to aid her navigate uncharted territories, including the unfamiliar medical field, her diagnosis, and her life moving forward. Eventually the palliative care team began asking Jean questions, including: where she was born (Kentucky), activities she had neglected but wanted to get back to (making soup for her family and doing chores like laundry), and ideas/beliefs she held near/dear to her heart.

After the initial visit the patient remained in close contact with each member of the palliative care team. She had monthly visits with her physician to review her medications and ensure that her pain was adequately controlled. In addition, the doctor also addressed any new medical issues and provided appropriate treatment. The social worker checked in with the patient a few times a week to ensure that she had access to all the resources she needed to accomplish her daily tasks. She also worked with the patient to formulate goals and direct her to support groups and websites for pancreatic cancer. Finally, the chaplain (an incredibly positive presence during the interactions) offered spiritual resources and assessed Jean's outlook on life and her thoughts on death. He also went some thoughts on potential bumps and strains that the patient could experience regarding her marriage.

Overall, I was very impressed with the care provided by the palliative care team with each delivering a separate assessment and plan for the patient and contributed to the goals of the group. The team was also extremely inviting/approachable and sought input from the patient's family members. For instance they asked the daughters what Jane's favorite activities were. When asked, the girls mentioned that their mom loved fishing. The team quickly responded with a planned family fishing trip to the local state park. The team also sensed Jane's fear of losing her independence and anxiety about her future and the upcoming changes in her life. Rather than question her directly, the team gathered input from other family members. Jane's husband was able to step in and articulate/identify the most profound changes in the patient's mood/behavior. In addition, he was able to list some of his favorite shared activities that had been disrupted by his wife's diagnosis.

Another aspect of palliative care is the personalized tailor-made plan constructed for each patient. There were multiple instances where the palliative team members pushed Jane to go outside her comfort zone, rather than put off events. On one occasion, Jane was considering skipping out on a school board related function to devote more time to her immediate family and dealing with her diagnosis. Jane discussed her thoughts on this with her social worker who quickly insisted that she go to the event because of its significance to her. On the flip side, the social worker also counseled Jane about her anxiety caused by an inability to hang out with friends. Jane noticed that the pain medications along with worsening fatigue, made it difficult to meet with all her former acquaintances daily which increased her anxiety. The palliative care team consoled her and explained that while some events, like the aforementioned school function, are still important to attend, other events like routine social meetings with friends may need to be postponed due to the physical toll of the drugs and cancer. This helped alleviate some of Jane's anxiety.

Discussing Jane's palliative care experience was enlightening. It's a relief to know that no matter what a patient's diagnosis, prognosis, or support system is, they have access to resources to better adapt and handle their situation. From a professional standpoint, it was refreshing to see so many disciplines come together to accomplish common goals. I especially liked the holistic approach seen in palliative care and I loved that all aspects of the patient's health: a) physical, b) mental, c) emotional, and d) spiritual were addressed. Having constant input from other friends/family was also beneficial to patient outcomes. I frequently see people struggle to manage their problems solely on their own.

Professionally, there were plenty of learning points from this palliative care case. First and foremost, I was refreshed on the precise definitions of palliative care, hospice care, and comfort care, along with the consultation process involved for each. I learned that pain/symptom control is just a small sliver of the services provided by the team. For Jane, the most valuable aspect of her palliative care team was the constant support and assistance with overcoming obstacles encountered when navigating the healthcare system. Moving forward with my medical career, I'll be sure to incorporate more holistic questioning and services. I'll ask more about family members, encourage input from spouses/children, explore patient's cultural and spiritual beliefs, and dive deeper into patient's internal motivations.

CHAPTER 7
Understanding the Patient's Addiction

CHASING TINA
KATE CLARK (MS 3 SEPTEMBER 2019)

On the third day of my psychiatry clerkship, we received a consult for a young woman, Tina (not her real name), who had been chased through the woods by aliens. She ran to her neighbors for help, who then took her to the hospital. She had been in the woods for an unknown period of time wearing only her underwear and was thus covered in small cuts, scrapes and insect bites. My psychiatry attending and I went down to the medical floor and asked her how she had come to be in the hospital. Tina seemed to find it difficult to focus on my attending's face, and although her speech was pressured and tangential, she was able to give us her story. While scratching her entire body uncontrollably, she said she had "done a bunch of meth," that she knew the aliens weren't real, that she was not going to take any medications, and that she needed to get home so she could pack her clothes and get everything in order to go to rehab. She was very emotionally labile, but redirectable and she remained relatively calm until she was told that she could not go home. Tina became very agitated, sat up quickly and started swinging her arms around, gesticulating wildly.

At this point, my heart rate quickened and I was trying not to look as terrified as I felt. My attending was still sitting calmly within Tina's reach as he explained why she needed to stay in the hospital and why she needed to begin taking medications. Tina began to curse loudly at my attending, calling him choice names for trying to fix her drug problem with more drugs and demanded that he leave her room. As we went out into the hallway and began to discuss the dopaminergic effects of methamphetamines on the brain, Tina stripped off her hospital gown, put on regular clothes and started down the hallway, muttering that she was going to leave this place and walk home. Tina passed all of the obvious exits, stairwells and elevators, wandered onto the opposite wing of the same floor, and hurried around corners anytime she noticed the nurses, me, or my attending following her. She disappeared in a hallway that ended in an emergency exit. She was found in an empty room with the lights off, hiding behind the door, holding a piece of paper over her head. Tina was frustrated to be found and began to wander off in a new direction. Hospital security then arrived and helped her back to her room. After further discussion, Tina was still agitated and unwilling to take any medications, so campus security had to restrain her as the nurse gave her a dose of IM Geodon.

A few days later, Tina was getting ready for discharge. She told me she remembered me from somewhere but couldn't place me. The clarity in her eyes and the change in her pattern of speech were in such stark contrast to that first day. Tina was very pleasant, laughing and apologizing for her previous behavior and telling us that her last time on meth had scared her so badly that she never wanted to take it again. She recalled seeing the aliens, but also told us that she had seen God during that episode, and He walked her through her life and mistakes. She left in good spirits, expressing her desire to get clean and get closer to God. She wished me good luck in school.

Tina took me out of my comfort zone. At first, she scared me. A patient under the influence of illicit substances can become physically aggressive, and I appreciated the way my attending modeled an approach that kept the situation under control. She was the first person I had ever seen who was acutely intoxicated on any sort of illicit substance and I had no idea how to navigate such an interaction. I was still a bit uncomfortable when I was sent to try to get more history the morning after the consult. She did not like to be asked the same questions over and over again, especially when I had no control over her situation or the ability to let her go home. I did not push her as much as I normally would due to witnessing her behavior the day before. Once she calmed down, I started to sympathize with her situation. She was trapped in an unfamiliar place, suffering from methamphetamine intoxication, itching uncontrollably, and simply wanting to sleep in her own bed. Most patients would rather not be in the hospital, regardless of the reason. Patients do not typically like to be awakened by medical students and asked numerous, repetitive questions. Yet, I have a responsibility to all of my patients to gather enough information to make informed decisions about their healthcare. Patients may not like me for it, but I will be providing the best health care I can. Tina was a bit of desensitization therapy for my fears of agitated patients and conflict. She pushed me one step closer to being as calm as my attending was while staring down an angry and threatening patient.

Tina's improvement during her stay and her determination to begin rehab was a nice reminder that people will sometimes gain the insight and motivation required to change their lives for the better. I do not want to be completely naïve and take everything patients tell me at face value, but I also do not want to become cynical or jaded towards every patient that says they will try lifestyle modification. Lifestyle changes, whether they are related to substance abuse or diet and exercise, are difficult to make, especially when complicated by addiction and dependence. As physicians, we cannot force patients to change their behaviors, but we must be supportive, even if they are attempting to change for the 50th time. It is easy to assume that people with substance use disorder want to be imprisoned by a drug, but it is much more difficult to see the person and their struggles and how they arrived at where they are now. Unrecognized biases place a wall between the patient and physician that does not allow a functional relationship to form. Tina left me with a lot to think about and several behaviors of my own to modify. I will continually search for and challenge my biases throughout medical school and my career to attempt to eliminate their negative effects on my patients' care.

A TOTAL SHIFT
CAITLAN JONES (CRS JULY 2020)

As most patients in the community health clinic in Western KY, Brenda (not her real name) has lived there since she was little. Her family still lives there, and they are a huge part of their life. Brenda is a 35-year-old female who is a recovering addict. She has three children ages 14, 16, and 18. The real kicker is that they are all boys. She was a sweet and very talkative lady with a hard exterior. An exterior that shields the common person from seeing her struggling past. Brenda is an alcoholic. She didn't realize the severity of her chronic alcoholism until a little over a month ago. After some heavy drinking and a near death experience, she found herself in the hospital and very, very sick. She quickly told me, "I hate hospitals". But it was a nine day stay in one that kept her alive and was the first steppingstone in turning her life around. After leaving the hospital and going through a detox period, she now lives with her mother and is trying to break her crippling habit. The years of abuse have taken a toll on her and she now has to take vitamin B12 supplements for the rest of her life. Considering the circumstances though, she enjoys living with her mom. Her mother was with her at this follow up appointment and her genuine concern and love for her daughter could not be denied. When Brenda was asked if she was very active, she said yes as she does a lot of yard work and helps out her grandmother often. She went on to explain that she spends a lot of time with her grandmother who currently lives nearby, just across the railroad tracks. She currently works at a local grocery and admitted that while she hasn't been completely sober, she drinks significantly less than she had. She didn't shy away from talking about her shortcoming in taking shots on occasion but instead was rather open. She had found an ally and supporter in Dr. S who allowed her to be honest so that they could set a realistic yet stern plan of care moving forward. Overall, she seemed happy even with dealing with all the anxiety and changes that have rapidly occurred in her life. And if I had to bet, I would bet there were several smiles behind that COVID forced face mask as a young woman was developing into a new normal.

This lady had abused alcohol for a really long time and Dr. S mentioned that even a small relapse could have large consequences. He was very real with her and told her that one bad night could kill her. They made a strategic plan to continue to cut down on her drinking and he didn't ignore how hard this change was for her. The biggest thing I noticed was how concerned her mom was. She had seen her baby girl go through a tragedy and just wanted her to do better, feel better, and be better. When her daughter admitted to drinking a few times this past month you could see her heart crumble into a million pieces and question if she had failed as a mother. Dr. S mentioned that her mom was with her at the last appointment and that the patient he saw this day was a completely different one from the one he saw right after the hospital stay. She was carrying conversations, staying focused, and dedicated to getting herself better. A total shift from before.

ALWAYS DO THE RIGHT THING
COLLIN MCGLONE (CRS JULY 2022)

H grew up in Kentucky. He has a caring mother and father, who taught him discipline, showed him love, and tried to bring him up right. He is close to his uncle, who was always there for him when he had a problem. Growing up, he developed a passion for the arts, and is interested in music and writing.

At home, H has a loving girlfriend and was just recently blessed with a daughter named A. Hayden has had some dark times in his life, but just as the moon lights up the night sky, A does that for him. He wants to provide everything for her, but she gives him hope as he goes through a rough patch in his life during his hospital stay.

H and his girlfriend work hard to make ends meet. Working a blue-collar job with bills to pay and a family to take care of, stress can compound. This stress combined with other factors ultimately led to his current hospital stay. Although it has been a difficult time for him, his daughter, his passion for writing, and the people in the hospital are getting him through, and he is feeling better already with big plans when he gets out.

Throughout his stay, H has been reading and writing to keep his mind occupied. After reading his poem to us he wrote for his daughter and some of his plans for a book he would like to write someday, it is clear that he is an empathetic and caring person. Calling it "America", he told us he wants to write about understanding others struggles and the tenets that he believes our generation of Americans has to keep in mind as they navigate life. He believes perspective, practice, and perseverance are keys to success and being a good person. In addition, H has plans to get educated. Once he gets better, he wants to look into applying to college and studying writing or music.

When asked what advice H would have for us as future doctors, it sounded as though this advice came straight from a practicing doctor or professor. He told us to be kind, be disciplined in our work, and follow the rules. But more importantly than rigidly following rules, always try to do the right thing. Most importantly, don't pursue this career for the wrong reasons – get to know patients, care for them, and pursue this because you want to save lives.

CAUSE AND EFFECT
ELIZABETH LYONS (PRE-MATRIC JUNE 2021)

Societal pressures emphasize the ideology of crammed schedules, showing strength over weakness, and being busy is better. However, what the world is beginning to see is the toll this lifestyle takes on the human body and mind. We have seen a growing focus on self-care and mental health, yet people are still held to the standard of performance determines a person's worth. The feeling of not being good enough, thinking no one cares, or a fear of failure are all common for many individuals. For one man, who says he's lost everything, these feelings are all too real. Here is his story of how his *then* led him to *now* desperately seeking for someone to listen and his search for *when* he'll find normalcy.

He grew up on a farm where his love of fishing and hunting formed. An active lifestyle was his normalcy, and now laid a foundation for the normal he longed to find again. Fishing to him was not solely a fun pastime, but symbolized the connection he held with his dad that grew stronger with time as he transitioned from childhood to adulthood. A lack of self-worth and confidence began to repeatedly surface as he quickly brushed past his time growing up. A high school drop-out who never felt good enough, found alcohol to just get by. Ten years ago he said his wife left because he drank too much, so a handful of pills seemed like the only option to permanently end the heartbreak he felt. From then on, alcohol began stripping away everything in his life.

The normalcy he desperately wants to find, will never again be attainable. He will never eat a solid meal again. Nightly programming and a plastic tube are the only means of nutrients he will receive. No hope for a transplant, no hope for any surgery because the surgeons say he would die on the table. The alcohol he thought would comfort him resulted in pancreatitis and chronic excruciating pain. He wanted to go to sleep and never wake up because he was so tired of the pain. He explained he could no longer work because the pain controlled him. A small printing business provides him with income and a sense of purpose, but that isn't good enough. His uncle constantly nags at him to move out of his grandmother's and find a job where he can by physically moving. Good days are an anomaly, but when the pain is less than usual, he hops on a boat to fish with his dad. He says the connection with his dad is still there, but the exertion causes him to bed ridden for weeks afterwards. What brings him the most joy results in debilitating pain. Again, something he once loved will never be the same. Physical pain is unbearable, but with medicine and rest it can be managed. For him, the hardest part is having no one who listens or cares because the alcohol pushed them away. When the pain becomes too much and his family pushes him aside, he turns back to alcohol to temporarily numb the pain.

Expectations and realities are two very different ideas. He longs to return to the man he once was, and never see what he says is a "shell of the man I was before" again. The reality is, the permanent feeding tube and crippling pain will never go away because surgery is no longer an option. He is seeking to find when he can return to normalcy, but sadly that day will just be an imaginative reality he won't be able to find.

We pursue a profession as physicians so we can heal and treat people. Today, I saw a side of medicine where a prescription or surgery won't "fix" the patient and quickly help them feel better. I saw patients leave as their nurses and doctors wondered if the next time their name appeared it would be on an obituary. The patient who shared his story had an alcohol addiction, and wanted to die because he didn't have any support. I wanted to fix his pain and broken relationships, but I couldn't. Dr. B shared advice with me that I will carry with me throughout the entirety of my life. He stated, "Our responsibility ends where our ability stops." Patients will die and some may never step foot back into your building, but we don't have the ability to control every scenario. Medicine is listening and showing compassion to each patient, an ability all physicians hold. Everyone just wants to know someone cares, and that may be the best healing of all.

HAPPY FATHER'S DAY
BRADLEY WATSON (PRE-MATRIC JUNE 2021)

Meeting by luck, intersecting in Western Kentucky, X's parents came from Ohio and California. Moving around and growing up in Kentucky and Georgia was challenging, but X felt it helped him grow. His childhood consisted of moving around and his parents split in a divorce during his childhood. After almost finishing high school in Georgia, he moved back to Western Kentucky where he felt it was always home.

Mr. X began working and met his future wife and married at a young age. She brought with her two kids from a previous relationship who he quickly took in as his own children. Along with these two stepchildren brought into his life, X had two additional children with his wife. X loved all his children very dearly and discussed how much they meant to him, and how hard he worked to make sure they were provided for in every way. However, Mr. X also discussed how his wife struggled with mental illness, often making trips to the psychiatrist to help with her struggles. This would place a strain on Mr. X, the kids, and their relationship, being the downfall of their relationship.

On Father's Day 2021, Mr. X was desperate to see his kids and prepared a day with them. However, fighting with his wife prior to the date made X's chances of seeing his kids feel impossible. Alcohol leading up to the day as well as on the day only fueled the fire that would quickly become violent. While drinking heavily, he began cutting his wrist in practice to commit suicide before finally making a large slice parallel with his forearm. Realizing what he did, he quickly called his friend in regret. Still intoxicated and unsure of his decision to receive help, X fought with his friends' urges to send him to the emergency department. Through a relentless effort, X's friend was able to place him into the care of the psychiatry unit where he was adamant about how amazing the care he had received was.

Mr. X is looking past his suicide attempt and is committed on getting better without using medicine. He believes therapy alone is a great place to start and doesn't want to rely on medicine in the event he has to come off of it. Recently X finished receiving his high school diploma and plans to get into a better line of work to provide for his children. He also plans to follow up with a psychiatrist regularly to learn new coping strategies and ways to reduce his stress level.

After talking with this patient, it changed my entire perspective on those within the psychiatric ward. Many people within this ward just have bad breaks or clouded judgement during a decision. I think by properly equipping these patients with coping strategies and ways to prevent stress within their lives, it can help prevent recurrences in patients' lives. It is also interesting to see how detrimental drug and alcohol usage can be for those with amplified emotions and create a situation which can easily lead to death.

KLONOPIN FOR A HIGH
TATE BURRIS (PRE-MATRIC JUNE 2021)

Mr. J is a middle-aged man who grew up in Western Kentucky. He lived his whole life there even after his parents and siblings left and moved away. He never went to college, and started doing odd jobs after he got out of high school. He did everything from construction to sanitation to lawn care, he said that he did it all. He bounced around between these jobs because he struggled with drug problems and kept failing drug tests and getting fired. With no family around he developed severe depression and anxiety and had constant panic attacks coupled with his problem with abusing drugs, this drove him to isolate himself from everyone. Recently both of his parents passed away and he moved to stay with his brother until they got everything figured out with the will for their parents. That was about six months ago and still nothing has been resolved with the will and his brother has kicked him out of his house because he refuses to pay anything, or help with anything around the house. He says he has been staying in his car for the last three weeks when he came in to see Dr. K about his depression and anxiety. He told Dr. K that the only thing that has ever helped was Klonopin but that he has only been able to get it from a friend because no doctor would prescribe him any because of his history of drug use. Once Dr. K said he was not going to prescribe him Klonopin and offered an alternative treatment, Mr. J stopped talking and refused to take the other medications, showing that he was only there to get the Klonopin so he could get a high, not deal with his depression and anxiety.

This man has lived a hard life no doubt, he didn't grow up with much, both of his parents have passed away, and his brother, the only family he has left, kicked him out and want's nothing to do with him. I can see where living this life could drive someone to do the things that this man did. All this considered, no reason is reason enough to abuse drugs. This man needs to get help outside of medication. Therapy, drug counseling, rehab, all of these are things that could be greatly beneficial to this man if he would do them, but sadly it does not seem like he is willing to. I've seen how drug addiction can affect a person, but I have also seen people get through it with hard work. I hope this man gets the help that he needs, but at the end of the day it is his decision if he wants the help or not.

LACK OF FORMAL EDUCATION AFFECTS HEALTH DECISIONS
SUMMER SPARKS (CRS JULY 2020)

Mrs. E is 71 years old. She is the youngest girl of 7 children. She fondly remembers walking to elementary school and buying butter for her mom at a corner grocery. When she was a teenager, she entertained herself by going to the roller-skating rink with her older sisters. Her father was employed in a meat packing plant, but his pay was in the form of meat. Her mother earned money to pay bills by taking in laundry for others. Mrs. E and her sisters were expected to help their mother.

Because her family was impoverished, she dropped out of school in 11th grade because someone stole her textbooks and her family could not afford to replace them. She began working in a factory making nylon socks. She met her future husband while working there as he was her supervisor. She was married at age 21 and had her first son. She learned to drive after the birth of her second son, 4 years later. Her husband was hard-working putting in 100 hours per week as a farmer. She waited 11 years before the birth of her daughter, Melissa. Her husband died of a sudden cardiovascular event leaving her widowed for the last 20 years. She continues to live alone but has had three long-term relationships since the death of her husband. These 3 men also have all died. She now keeps the company of a small dog. Even as an elder, she says that she tries to keep up with latest fashion trends and loves to sew. She also attends dances every Saturday night at the local senior citizen dance hall. She is committed to her church family of 40 years. She participates in the choir and on the kitchen committee.

Mrs. E says that because she had very little education, she lacked crucial information about how to care for her body and make health-conscious decisions. Today, she suffers from various health issues that could have been prevented if only she had known how her lifestyle decisions could affect her future health. Mrs. E began smoking cigarettes when she was 15 years old. She was influenced by her older sisters who also smoked. Because nicotine is so addictive, she is still a current smoker. She currently has been diagnosed with Chronic Obstructive Pulmonary Disease (COPD) and hypertension. Her chronic bronchitis causes shortness of breath and persistent coughing. She is already quite incapacitated with this long-term effect of smoking. It sometimes inhibits her from enjoying her hobby of dancing and babysitting her grandchildren. She has had numerous hospitalizations because of breathing issues. She is in the office today requesting new resources to help her with smoking cessation.

Mrs. E is optimistic about her future and anticipates her annual trip to Branson with her sister. She is motivated to improve her health status for the benefit of her family. She aspires to attend her last grandson's high school graduation.

Patient outcomes are more heavily reliant on support systems than I originally thought. It is important that one feels motivated to improve one's health, and many patients are encouraged by their loving families. I think that Mrs. E is attempting to set a good example for her grandchildren and children and wants to lead a heathy and responsible life. I think that it is common that many patients with poor social support are not as willing as Mrs. E to sacrifice their lifestyles and habits for their loved ones. I think that it is imperative for a physician to understand his or her patients' social incentives for wanting to improve their health. This is usually easier for rural physicians because they are usually responsible for seeing many generations of the same families.

MOM'S NEW BOYFRIEND WILL NEVER BE MY DAD TATE BURRIS (PRE-MATRIC JUNE 2021)

Mr. T is a 19-year-old male who currently lives in Western Kentucky. He hasn't always lived there though, throughout his childhood him and his family moved over eight times to different areas of Western Kentucky due to financial issues, and his dad bouncing around jobs. He lived with his mom, dad, and brother, and says that he had a wonderful childhood. His family was very close but he says that he and his dad were inseparable. They did everything together from hike, to fish, to play sports. He kept emphasizing the fact that his dad was his best friend. He said that he had a perfectly happy childhood up until the age of eight years old. It was at this time when he was sexually molested by his older male cousin. He said that ever since then he has always been on edge and looking over his shoulder and never trusting anybody. He explained that ever since then he began to shut people out and felt like the only person he could go to or trust was his dad.

It was shortly after this when Mr. T and his family moved where they would settle down for the foreseeable future. He attended school there all the way until he finished high school. It was during this time though that things really started going downhill for Mr. T. At around the age of 12 his dad started having some serious renal insufficiencies, around 15 his dad went into a stage of near complete renal failure, and when Mr. T was 17 his father passed away from both renal failure and congestive heart failure. During this whole time of his dad being sick, Mr. T had to take on more of the adult male figure in his house because his dad wasn't able to do the majority of the things he was able to do before. Mr. T was having to take care of his mom as well as his dad, on top of that he was no longer able to do all of the activities with his dad that he loved to do. This sent him into a pretty deep depressed state and because of this he started turning to drugs and alcohol.

After his dad's death, Mr. T began to slip deeper and deeper into a depressed state and kept experimenting with drugs and alcohol until he tried to take his life. He attempted to overdose but it did not work. He said that he regretted trying as soon as he did and went out to seek help. He said that he was doing better for a while until here recently when his mom began dating a new guy. He said that he had no problems with this man, and he was thankful that he made his mom happy, but the man began to try and act like a father figure to Mr. T. This sent him spiraling again. He started going back to drugs and alcohol, and a few days ago tried to overdose again. This attempt again did not work, and his mother had him admitted to the hospital for help.

In reflecting on my talk with Mr. T, I was heartbroken to hear what all he had been through in his life. In nineteen years, this man has been through more than most people will go through in their lives. Even though there is no good excuse to try and take your own life, I can understand why he was thinking the way that he did. The fact that after all of this he is actively trying to seek help is amazing. I could tell that he was hurting, but he was willing to get help, and I found that amazing.

MOONLIGHT PSYCHOSIS
NIKKI HARNAGE (CRS JULY 2022)

As we traded polite introductions, his eyes lit up when he learned we are close in age. His ensuing handshake was gentle, yet firm. Moving to the secluded (although observed) conference room, he ironically sat in the rolling office chair as I took a cushioned hospital chair. We shared a quick laugh about the reversal of roles.

I began, "This is your story. Share whatever you would like, whatever is important to you or to who you are."

He asked to run to his room to grab something. He returned with a classic, black composition notebook. As he flipped through the first few sheets, I noticed the pages were filled with neat, fat writing in colorful ink. He began to read; he had already written his story. He spoke of late nights taking care of family and described the stress that accompanied the endless hard work and sacrifices. He admitted turning to weed to escape and recounted the night that his escapism turned into a nightmare: feeling alone, and yet surrounded, he slipped out to the back porch to watch the moon light the sky. A retreat where he often found hope. Then, after a not-so-unusual blunt, he returned inside to his girlfriend and newborn daughter. He began to hear voices plotting against life while he lay in bed. As his paranoia worsened, he drove to the nearby gas-station. Eventually, he was admitted to the hospital and subsequently to the inpatient psych-ward.

While that page was dedicated to his past, the rest were devoted to his future. He dreamed of attending the local university to explore music and improve his writing. Further, he dreamed of publishing his work. With tears in his eyes, he shared another page deeper in the notebook. He spoke of his new daughter, the person that brightened his darkest moments as the moon did on many previous nights. He expressed how his devotion to family impossibly deepened upon her arrival and of how he wanted to be the father that everyone deserved. He said the best dads were the ones that freely disciplined and loved their children. In that moment, he also advised that the finest doctors were motivated by passion, kind, self-disciplined, malleable, and took the time to know their patient.

Upon exploring the idea of how to be a better self, he introduced his idea for another work to publish. He flipped his notebook to another page and spiritedly listed the outline on his fingers. Firstly, he imagined a reinvented America, defined by a unified empathy between its people, rather than geography. To walk a mile in another's shoes was not enough, but differences should more largely be set aside to learn from others. In doing so, the perspective, compassion, and empathy needed for change could redefine the current cultural landscape. Beyond this, however, he described how the deeply rooted American dream should be revived. While choosing hard work is not a comfortable decision, preparation and practice are the keys to success. In this aspect, and being a basketball fan, he particularly looked to Kobe Bryant as a role model. Further, such a work ethic should be accompanied by perseverance.

THE WARRIOR TATTOO
NITA NAIR (PRE-MATRIC JUNE 2021)

I met Hannah (not her real name) in the psychiatric ward on a hot, summer day. She was a sturdy, tattooed girl with a buzz cut, and the same age as me. I sat down with her to ask her about her life. She was friendly and more than happy to share her experiences. This is her story.

I asked Hannah an open-ended question about her childhood and she immediately jumped to the rough parts. I learned that her dad was an alcoholic who was abusive to her mother and her. When Hannah turned thirteen years old, she was raped for the first time. She was too scared to report the perpetrator, and turned to drugs and alcohol after the incident. In school, Hannah had issues with fitting in and was picked on often. She did not have much of a support system at that time, since her father had passed away from a heart attack and her mother was in and out of jail. Hannah was eventually placed in state's care around the age of fifteen. She wanted to live with her brother M, but was not allowed to because of his drug addiction. While she was under state's care, she would often run away and come back high from a medley of substances.

At the age of eighteen, Hannah returned to live with her mother after she was released from jail. One year later, she was raped for a second time. She was happy to hear that the man who raped her had been sent to prison after the police found a picture of a naked nine-year old on his phone.

Hannah then opened up to me about her experience of being in and out of recovery facilities. She talked about her struggles with suicidal thoughts. Hannah was eventually diagnosed with PTSD, bipolar disorder, and "a few other ones." She said she is learning how to accept the trauma, and is taking it one day at a time. Hannah hopes to get a sponsor soon and join Narcotics Anonymous. Along with her mental illnesses, Hannah also struggles with diabetes and wants to take control of her blood sugar. She strives to have a clearer mind and healthier body overall.

I asked Hannah to tell me about the moments in her life that make her smile. She briefly talked about journaling, coloring, and going to church, but spent most of her time talking about B, her orange cat with a floppy ear. She vividly remembers a time when she snuggled up with him as he purred and lifted his leg for belly rubs – a time when she forgot about everything else in the world. Hannah then talked to me about her love of animals and how she used to take care of horses. When her blood sugar allows her to, she loves horseback riding. She hopes to do that again soon.

I asked Hannah what she wants for her future. She paused for a while, as if she had not given this question much thought before. She then told me that wants to work with horses, be self-sufficient, make new friends and help others. Most of all she wants to be herself, and not try to be what others want her to be.

Though Hannah and I have had vastly different life experiences, I realized that we were not all that different. We both have similar desires for our futures – desires that are emphatically human. It was saddening to hear that Hannah's journey to her goals has been rougher than most. But I believe she will continue to persevere, as the warrior tattoo on her left arm suggests.

QUITTING IS HARD
CAITLAN JONES (PRE-CLINICAL JULY 2022)

"What's the hardest thing about quitting smoking?"

"Well first, you have to want to." JD told me this while talking about his lifetime love of cigarettes. I met JD while he was inpatient for COPD Exacerbation, Heart Failure Exacerbation, and Pneumonia. Some would call him strong-willed; others would call him stubborn. He's had an interesting life, one that has shaped who he is today and what kind of care he desires.

JD is a 71-year-old male who grew up in Eastern Kentucky. He was raised by his grandma. When he was 18, he decided to move to Dayton Ohio since there was nowhere to work in Eastern Kentucky. His biological mom lived in Dayton so that's where he found himself, and there he met his now wife, ND. They celebrated their 60th wedding anniversary last week.

JD said his wife is the best doctor he has ever had. She was with him in at the hospital and has been by his side over the years. She knows his medications and pays careful attention to his plan of care. They have 9 kids, 5 biological and 4 they adopted out of foster care. When raising their kids, JD built their dream house in Illinois from the ground up. But once they all graduated high school, they decided $6,000 a year in Illinois property tax wasn't fun and moved back to Kentucky; something JD had always wanted to do. Now, he is retired, but thinks fondly of his past career, helping distribute everything from magazines to junk mail.

JD has had COPD for about 30 years. His wife says he doesn't understand the severity of his disease and hasn't wanted to stop smoking. But no one has taken the time to explain to him exactly what COPD is. A few months ago, he had some bleeding ulcers and stomach surgery. He says ever since then he has been sick and weak. He's lost 50 pounds.

He quickly picked up my thick, rural Kentucky accent and I could tell he appreciated it. He was interested in where I was from and my voice alone helped build trust. He missed traditional medicine where your family doctor did all aspects of care from delivering babies to rounding in the hospital. His wife said, "There's a doctor for every part of your body, and when you get to the hospital no one is a familiar face". He doesn't like being in the hospital, he wants to go home very badly. Tomorrow morning he's going home, whether the doctors want him to or not.

JD is positive though, and he enjoys life. He said you can't stop from dying but you can decide to still have fun or to live in misery. When I asked what he wished his care team knew about him, he said "nothing really", he already tells them what he thinks. And he does. He's a funny, honestly blunt character. We talked about smoking, how it was relaxing and passed the time. He recalled a friend he helped stop drinking, but once JD moved to KY his friend started drinking again and died in his 40s as a result. He knows he needs to stop smoking and wants to cut back, but it's hard. It has been a part of his entire life starting when as a kid he picked up his dad's cigarettes buds.

He'll go home tomorrow, even if he shouldn't, and he probably will cut back on cigarettes. But I doubt he ever stops. This week was the first time he has ever truly wanted to do something about smoking, and in his words that's the hardest part.

ROAD TO RECOVERY
LAUREN TROUT (CRS JULY 2022)

From birth she has felt alone and that something is missing partly because she lost her twin sister in the womb due to a mother battling addiction while pregnant. Her childhood was laced with severe sexual, mental, and emotional abuse which she claims led to her history of cutting and alcohol/drug abuse. Later in her life, she received a Pell Grant to attend Stanford University online to get her forensics degree. With this degree, she worked in forensics online for a while. She was admitted to Psych because of her methamphetamine usage, and she is working hard to get off it and stay sober- she has been sober from drugs and alcohol for 2 weeks now. She is also officially 3 years clean of cutting and very proud of herself even though she admits that sometimes it is very hard to resist it, but she finds a way to fight it so that she can continue to be proud of herself. Something that brings her joy amid the darkness is her painting. She enjoys painting images of koi fish, clowns, and superheroes/villains. Upon getting discharged, she believes that this time will be different because she is willing to work hard to stay clean/sober and wants more stability in her life. She plans on going to rehab after being discharged to help her through her sobriety journey. As far as stability goes, she admits that she does not have a stable family so she will have to find stability in other aspects of her life. She is looking forward to reconnecting and getting to love on her puppy A when she leaves and having him as her companion during her recovery journey.

SELF-MEDICATING AFTER MY HUSBAND'S DEATH
SUMMER SPARKS (PRE-MATRIC JUNE 2021)

Ms. S is 62-year-old women from Western Kentucky. She is currently in the inpatient psychiatric facility. Upon asking the patient about her life's story, she describes her life as being blessed despite the fact that she has experienced great tragedy. Her story begins in her early childhood. She is the oldest daughter of a coal miner and a housewife. She has four younger siblings. Ms. S emphasizes that this part of her life was stable, and she felt very much like a normal child. However, when she was 11, her father was killed unexpectedly in a coal mining accident. She acknowledges that this event was traumatic for her because she was very close with her father, and she was old enough to fully understand what had transpired. This negatively affected her emotionally and also damaged the stability of her family. After her father died, her grief-stricken mother began to express a variety of negative attitudes and actions. Her mother developed a drinking habit, and she would frequently invite male suitors into the family's home. Ms. S explains that this made her feel angry and neglected. At age 13, Ms. S was raped by a man that had been invited over by her mother. This incident persuaded Ms. S to leave. She dropped out of 8th grade, and she married a boy she had met earlier when she was 14.

She described her marriage as very happy, and she and her husband had 2 children. She was married for forty-two years. Her husband passed away from cancer. When her husband died, she moved in with her son. She struggled intensely with the death of her husband and developed depression. Her son, who regularly used drugs such as methamphetamine, convinced her to experiment with drugs to help her sadness. In efforts to self-medicate, Ms. S developed a drug addiction. Last year, her son died from a drug overdose. She states that his death has been difficult to cope with because she has never truly lived on her own. She explained that she is voluntary admitted because she has recently been struggling with suicidal ideation. She has been here for 2 weeks.

Ms. S hopes to go live with her daughter when she leaves the hospital. She has been greatly encouraged to stop her drug use and seek help. She says that she has no other health issues, but she wants to be healthier so that she can be in her grandchildren's lives. She also intends on partaking in hobbies that she enjoys such as going to the movies and working in her vegetable garden.

SHARING A SMILE
DREW DODDS (PRE-MATRIC JUNE 2021)

Patient M is a mid-20s female who was born and raised on the Kentucky-Tennessee border. M is currently living in Western Kentucky. She has a 4-year-old son who she loves dearly and is spending a lot of time with his maternal grandmother. He loves ride-on-toys while Patient M enjoys walking outside, especially in the woods. Patient M and her son love to play in the wood chip pile at the back of the tobacco barn in addition to riding the 4-wheeler and golf cart.

Patient M attended school until half way through 12th grade as she no longer felt that high school was the environment for her. She ran Cross Country and wanted to try tennis but never had the time to start. She had a passion for basketball but when she didn't make the team due to a sports physical mix-up, she was able to join the team as their manager and participate in that capacity. Patient M has been to the lake but is scared of water moccasins and therefore doesn't enjoy it anymore and hasn't been back recently.

Patient M has been working on her addiction to alcohol and drugs for several years now. Her worst fears are wasps and bees and specifically being stung by one. Patient M also does not like lady bugs because when they fly, they appear to be similar to wasps and bees which invokes a large amount of unneeded stress.

Patient M has an awesome plan for the future. Her ideal future doesn't have to do with anything besides gaining full custody back of her son, becoming the best mom he could ever ask for. She would love to continue sharing her story and also sharing her smile to those around her. She would like to continue sharing her testimony specifically to younger people who are following the same paths and hopefully impact their lives in a positive way to stop these addictions. Patient M's smile seemed to be one to light up the room, no matter what is being discussed, which is a very admirable trait than many desire.

THAT WASN'T METH
HANNAH MARSHALL (CRS JULY 2020)

T was a thirty-year-old mother who had recently been admitted to the psych ward for visual and auditory hallucinations, suicidal ideation, and depression. She revealed that she had previously been admitted for suicidal attempts in the past as well as depression. She had been diagnosed with bipolar one disorder and had been off meth for a year. However, the night before she was admitted she took what she thought was meth, but after a tox screen in the ER it revealed she had benzos in her system.

She faults her auditory and visual hallucinations on the drugs and during our conversation she revealed she no longer had visual hallucinations, but often heard voices that would tell her "she wasn't good enough" or "the world would be better off without her in it".

T has two kids, both of which are in foster care, and is recently widowed. She revealed that her husband passed away within the last few months. She described how it led her into a depressive episode, which typically last 3-4 weeks, which in turn lead her to relapse on drugs. T is very upset and disappointed that she relapsed because she had been working to get her kids back in her custody and to be a better mother.

T revealed more regarding her disease to me further in our conversation. She revealed that in her manic episodes she had moments of impulsive purchasing, grandiose feelings, and loss of sleep. These episodes usually only lasted a week or two and were typically followed by three to four weeks of depressive episodes which included: increased fatigue/sleep, suicidal ideation, and feelings of regret from her manic episodes.

When talking with T it is clear that she is goal oriented. She brought herself to the ER from a rehab facility to seek help for management of her bipolar disorder. She reveals that she was in a very low place and was afraid she may hurt herself if she hadn't come in. She wants to participate in group therapy to learn coping mechanisms to deal with the loss of her husband and children as well as mechanisms to help her cope with her depressive episodes and suicidal thoughts.

Talking with T didn't make me feel uncomfortable or afraid like I previously thought I would. I realized that T was just an individual who was dealing with dense life events and needed help. After being on the psych floor it is clear that mental health and mental disorders are just like any other physical ailment that needs to be treated or managed. A broken bone, heart failure or back pain is no different from bipolar disorder or depression. These are all "ailments" that people experience and as a physician it is our responsibility to help individuals manage it.

THE RECOVERED ADDICT WITH A COMPLICATED FAMILY DYNAMIC
KENNEDY BREEDING (PRE-MATRIC JUNE 2020)

As I stood outside of the exam room, the resident I was following for the day handed me the nurse intake note of a patient waiting on the other side of the door. Looking at the notes, I gathered that Ms. P, a 52-year-old female with high blood pressure, was waiting on the other side. An odd sense of anticipation rose up in my stomach as I prepared to go in and interview her. Her papers gave me her height, weight, allergies and a laundry list of other things to note, but soon I would be asking her personal history questions that could be just as important.

Opening the door to exam room four, I saw a woman of short stature wearing sweatpants and a t-shirt, waiting anxiously on the edge of the exam table. As I introduced myself and asked if she would be willing to participate in an interview while she waited for the doctor to come in, she nodded and told me to go right ahead. The first question was simple enough, "So tell me about your life," I said with the routine rhythm I had picked up from weeks of conducting similar interviews. "Oh boy!" she said as she rolled her eyes. "Where do I even start?" Ms. P then began to describe her childhood. She explained that she grew up with a sister and a brother and that her parents raised them to be hard workers. "I've always worked. While other kids in my class were going to Disney World, I was stuck at home working to pay for my school shoes." She also explained that her father, a WWII MP, expected a sense of order in the household. This definitely showed his children's work ethic. This work ethic is what went on to push Ms. P through difficult times, she explained. "I had my first daughter while I was still in high school but I still graduated on time.", she said with pride.

Following her high school graduation, Ms. P experienced more hardships. Her brother passed away due to kidney disease and her mother passed away just 21 days after the passing of her brother. However, Ms. P stayed busy raising three children, two daughters and one son. She then explained that sometime after the death of her mother, she got mixed up in the wrong crowd and became addicted to drugs. "I thought I was cute, but now I am paying the price for it at 52." Though she has been clean for some time now, the effects of her addiction are still present. Her eldest daughter became a heroin addict but after Ms.P's daughter lost her two children in what she called "a big wakeup call", she used suboxone to get clean and has since regained custody of the children. Ms. P says that she doesn't get to see them too much since they live several hours away but talks to them on the phone frequently.

Ms. P also took the time to explain her complicated family dynamic. Her son, an openly gay man living in another part of the state, no longer talks to the rest of the family after a fight that ended when he used derogatory terms to describe Ms.P's youngest biracial daughter. After that Ms.P used another derogatory term to describe him and the two haven't spoken since. Ms.P remains close to her youngest daughter who still lives in the area. "We look nothing alike but we act the same way!" she explains with a chuckle. Ms.P also explained that she is really close to the daughter of her youngest daughter. "She actually wanted to come and visit with me today but I'm too anxious about these results." she said as she once again went into her family's history of poor health and battles with high blood pressure, cancer and heart disease. "I should have gotten this checked out way sooner but I kept putting it off."

When I asked Ms.P about her ideal future, she responded. "I just want to be able to relax with no one bothering me, but I guess that's part of life" with a shrug. After thanking Ms.P for the time, I left to go get the resident scheduled to see her. As I shut the door, I left Ms.P alone for probably the only 5 minutes she would get to herself all day. Though it's probably not what she had in mind, I hoped it allowed her to find some sort of peace and quiet even if it was in a busy clinic with the halls outside buzzing with nurses, patients and doctors.

WHAT CAN CURE MY DEPRESSION?
JOHN DAVIS (PRE-MATRIC JUNE 2022)

Mr. G's story begins in the pacific northeast. He was born in Washington state, and shortly after, he moved to Oregon where he was raised up until graduation of high school. He decided to enlist in the military upon graduation. More specifically, he decided to keep it close to the water by choosing the Navy. He served a few years, and eventually left the service sometime in the late 1990s. He since has had an issue with homelessness and ended up in Western Kentucky.

Mr. G admits that his memory is quite jaded due to over 20 overdoses from drug abuse in conjunction with longstanding depression and suicidal ideation he has battled since the age of 17. He states he has tried nearly every antidepressant medication, therapy, and combination there is, but still just isn't able to get rid of his depression and it has left him practically uninterested in everything. Outside of his own personal care, he has one biological daughter and 3 stepchildren which he feels some responsibility to care for and are "lots to take care of." As for things that do provide him some sense of joy, he enjoys listening to music and has plans to pick up where he left off with learning the guitar upon discharge from the hospital. He knows the beginning of the opening riff to "Smoke on the Water", and I think he will have no problem mastering the complete riff soon.

WHERE IS THE LIGHT AT THE END OF THE TUNNEL? TATE BURRIS (CRS JULY 2020)

Mr. C is a 55-year-old man who grew up in Western Kentucky with his mom, dad, four sisters and five brothers. His dad has passed away as well as two of his sisters and two of his brothers. He went to high school in an adjoining county where he played football and basketball until the tenth grade when he dropped out so he could work to help his mom with financial support. He worked at a farming supply store for 17 years until he got married and had a son. After he was married, he moved to Indiana where his wife had a job lined up. He lived there for two years until he got divorced and then moved back to Western Kentucky where he began working construction. He did this for a few more years until his mother got real sick and his sister had a stroke so he quit so he could focus all of his time on taking care of them. Throughout all of this time he struggled with heavy alcohol and drug use. This combined with his traumatic life situation led to him becoming very depressed and suicidal. He even climbed onto the side of a bridge and had every intention to jump until a police officer stopped him. He got help after this, and said that he was doing better until his son passed away last year. This led to him getting back on alcohol and drugs and drove him to put a knife to his throat in front of his sick mother. He decided not to and instead admitted himself to the behavioral health floor at the hospital where he says that he is felling a lot better.

Hearing everything that this man has been through in his life made me so sad. I could not imagine living the life he has. He has been through so many traumatic experiences that it is completely understandable that he feels depressed and suicidal. It is so hard to look at life in a positive light when you have only seen negativity for so long, and that is where this man is. But even though he has been through so much, he is still actively searching for ways to be better. It says a lot about him that when times were tough, he decided to go to the behavioral health department for help instead of actually killing himself. I think that is because he doesn't want to leave his mom and sister because they still need him, and I love that. The fact that he is willing to do whatever he needs to do to get help so that he can be the best for his mom and sister is just touching to me.

STATE GUARDIAN
COLLIN MCGLONE (PRE-MATRIC JUNE 2023)

Jim (not his real name) was tall and bearded man with a firm handshake and a pleasant affect. He spoke with a southern twang and smiled often, but he was reserved. Over the course of our interview, I learned a lot about him.

Jim was born 29 years ago in Western Kentucky. His parents split up while he was very young. Things got messy sometimes and his father was not always around, but he spent time between them, and it was alright. He enjoyed being outside and living in the country, and always liked to ride four wheelers with his friends. He also enjoyed basketball and began playing that at an early age. He made two friends during these years that he would keep into his adult life.

As Jim became a man, he began working in restaurants for some time, and some various construction jobs which he enjoys. He still enjoys basketball and riding four wheelers and engages in those activities when he gets the chance. He is a fanatic for UK basketball, and he is hoping UK gets another championship soon. He doesn't have much family here and hasn't started a family of his own, but he has made some friends.

Some of the friends Jim made were not the best of influences, unfortunately. He got into some risky behavior and drugs, and the outcome was detrimental. He spent some time incarcerated and was required to have a state guardian.

Jim is no longer using drugs and has moved on from this, but his guardian requires him to live at an assisted living facility. This is what led him to where he is now. He is clean and wants another go at living right, but he has trouble being excited for the future when he cannot leave the facility, and he says many of the hopeless people in the facility with him make him depressed and feel hopeless himself. This depression is what makes him concerned, and he is trying to get it under control.

When he can see a positive future, he envisions himself getting his own place, and maybe working with his enjoyment of operating equipment as a forklift operator. He wants to move back to where his family lives and to be near the lake. He is striving towards this goal by trying to change his outlook and keeping his mind busy while in a less than optimal situation. His advice to me as a future doctor was to keep an open mind and open ears so I can hear what my patients say and give good feedback that helps them get to a better place.

While speaking with Jim, I could not understand how he ended up in his current situation, where he lacks full autonomy, at less than a decade older than myself. I believe he must have grown a great deal from the person he was when placed under state guardianship. Jim was hesitant to share some details of his life, but I hoped he really was doing as good as he seemed, and I hope he reaches his goal.

TALK LESS, LISTEN MORE
BRIAN HART (PRE-MATRIC JUNE 2023)

I had the good privilege to speak to one of the patients, who I'll call "T," in the psychiatric ward today. While our conversation included facts related to her diagnoses and mental health, in general, its focus was the things that usually won't be found on any EHR chart. It mainly focused on the things that make patient T human.

A few simple things about T: Her favorite meal would consist of watermelon, pizza, fried squash (specifically, breaded with cornmeal and lemon pepper), and a Mountain Dew. Her favorite colors are red and black. She said that she feels like that combination matches her personality. T always thought of getting a tattoo of a girl at a vanity, surrounded by drugs, looking in the mirror at a red and black demon. Not surprisingly, T said she feels like that's the most accurate reflection of how she feels about herself – despite her belief in a deity that loves her unconditionally.

Outside the psychiatric ward, T has a German shepherd/ husky mixed-breed dog. She also has a cat. In addition to her younger half-sister, who she's really close to, T's mom is also still alive, and they have a good relationship, too. T also has an older brother and four older half-sisters, but she isn't as close to any of these because they are not local – spread out from Louisville to North Carolina. Her dad is dead; he died manufacturing methamphetamines. She was never as close to him because of this and the fact that he was constantly in and out of prison. In addition to the family members that she has strong ties to, T's support system consists of her ex-boyfriend; her current girlfriend, K and her best friend, E. She likes to go hiking with E and likes to play board games with K and K's daughter. Unfortunately, T doesn't have much time for hobbies with these folks, or by herself, though, since she holds down two jobs to make ends meet – one, as a team lead at the meat-packing plant and the other, as a back line cook at fast food.

T says that her support system will probably be a little disappointed and maybe somewhat angry that she has relapsed and found herself in the psychiatric ward again, but they will quickly get over it and be supportive of her. She is concerned that the rest of her family, though – her grandmother and cousins, especially – will have all sorts of judgmental opinions they won't hesitate to share, and that distresses her. She's almost certain that she will hear her grandmother angrily yell at her. When I asked why she thought this, T replied, "Simple. Because she's always angrily yelling at me." Not exactly the picture of fresh-baked cookies and holiday dinners that I think comes to mind for most of us when we think of grandma.

When I asked about her childhood, T shared that her first exposure to the alcohol she would later abuse, was when she was two years old, when she got drunk from beer cans laying around the house. Her exposure to the idea of drugs, especially methamphetamines, came around the first and second grade, when she distinctly remembers peeking under the door to her mother and father's bedroom begging them to come out and spend time with her and her siblings, instead of staying in and getting high. She wouldn't see them for several hours after having begged for their company. Her family moved around a lot until she was in the fifth grade, when they moved into a trailer park in Indiana.

She had a troubled time through school and ended up getting expelled from her high school, even though she got her GED shortly after getting expelled. She didn't care for school because of the structure and because nobody seemed to understand her. She did recall one class, though – home economics – that she says she didn't really like, except for the teacher, who always treated her respectfully "and like an actual person."

It's been four years since her federal felony gun charges came down, and her opportunities are still limited by the specter that casts over her. She still has dreams, though. T hopes to one day request a pardon for her felony and go back to school to become a nurse working in a psychiatric ward – helping others like herself. By that time, she hopes to still be with her girlfriend, with a child of her own – which she says she envisions probably having to be by artificial insemination, since felons can't generally adopt. She would want to live in a suburban house – somewhat isolated, but not too far from the amenities of city life – with the family she'll start with K, instead of being alone, in a cramped apartment, where when it gets dark, her only option is to be afraid alone. More than anything, though, her hopes for the future are to be at peace, without the worries and stress from her past to weigh her down.

I asked T what advice she had for somebody at the beginning of the journey towards becoming a doctor, regarding how to be the best type of doctor. "Simple. Talk less, listen more." T says none of her doctors have ever asked her questions like this before; they only see the chart and her diagnoses, from which they throw medicines at her without explanation, and "put words in [her] mouth" about her thoughts, feelings, and actions – which she says are rarely true – just to match what they see on the chart.

We're not taught to ask these questions as medical professionals, but there was pretty clear therapeutic value to T from my having slowed down to ask her about these things, and honestly, it was therapeutic to me, too. As someone about to start the process of becoming a doctor, having someone in such invisible anguish acknowledge that this is the type of conversation that needs to happen more often has left a distinct and lasting impression on me. While the specifics of her story are hers, realizing that there are common threads between us – as simple as that patients like T also have pets – helps me to see patients as more than just problems to be solved, but as people to be valued and respected, too.

ALONE IN A CROWDED ROOM
COLE WELLS (CRS JULY 2023)

"Sometimes you can feel alone in a crowded room." This is how he described to me he was feeling as we observed the hustle and bustle of the in-patient psych ward. "Would you mind sharing your story with me?" I ask him inquisitively. "I'm so happy you asked", he responded. "Okay great, tell me about anything you would like."

He began by sharing the haunting experiences of his early childhood and what ultimately led him to where he is today. With an abusive father growing up, he never felt safe within the confines of his home. Seeking refuge, he found himself living down the street at his grandparents' house. This was a much better situation for him despite the fact that he felt as if they were adding to his burden by pushing their religious views onto him. To ease the pain, he began experimenting with substances at the tender age of thirteen. With tears welling in my eyes, we locked gazes which revealed to me the depth of his pain. We took a moment to pause before I decided to inquire about any glimmers of happiness he remembers growing up. "I finally felt some relief from everything going on at home when I started seeing my current girlfriend. We've been dating off and on ever since the first day we met". Unfortunately, his girlfriend was also struggling with substance abuse which only intertwined their struggles. One night, they decided to take a pill they assumed to be a pain reliever and found out later that it was laced with fentanyl. With fear in his voice, he screamed for help and frantically tried to find the Narcan they had in case of an emergency. He doesn't remember much more from that night, but described waking up in the hospital the next morning thanking God that his girlfriend was still alive. Upon discharge, he began stealing from friends and family in order to feed their habit. This led to him stealing a car and ultimately getting charged with grand theft auto. In a last-ditch effort to escape his prison sentence, he decided to attend a court ordered faith-based rehabilitation group. This unfortunately did not live up to his expectations and he found himself left with suicidal idealizations. I could hear his struggle as he tried to get out the next sentence. "I tried to commit suicide a few days later." I looked deep into his eyes and told him how glad I was that he was sitting in front of me today.

As his story came to end, I saw a spark in his eyes which was a testament to the transformation he had undergone. "Thank you for allowing me to share my story without passing judgment." In this moment, I realized by lending a compassionate ear, I had truly made a difference in his life, and he had made a difference in mine.

CHAPTER 8

Curiosity Animates Empathy

A CURIOUS REFLECTION
BILL CRUMP, MD

I recently received an invitation to provide a reflection at the beginning of our hospital medical staff meeting. Having attended these quarterly meetings in person with my colleagues while sharing an outstanding meal for almost 25 years, I had appreciated the short prayers and poems. We even had an a cappella rendition of an inspirational hymn one time. To engage attendees via zoom, I considered what a group of physicians and other providers who are giving up some of their evening for a meeting might appreciate. I decided that since we talk a lot about the Triple Aim in medicine, but less about the importance of physician satisfaction as the fourth element, that would be the topic of my five-minute reflection.

My perspective on this issue is framed by the last eight years of our longitudinal study of changes in empathy and burnout among our medical students and residents. As we reviewed the literature, the definition for empathy that fits best for us is a true understanding of what it's like to be that patient. When a new diagnosis or a new medication or intervention is considered, how will it fit into the life of the individual in our exam room with us? In this sense, empathy is a cognitive function and significantly different from the emotional aspects of feeling sympathy, which is something else. The literature is also clear that physicians with higher measured empathy not only have better patient outcomes and more satisfied patients, but they are happier themselves and report lower levels of burnout. Studies of group physician practices show there are three elements that predict higher physician satisfaction and lower burnout. These are a personal sense of autonomy, agency, and meaning. Autonomy simply means that one has some influence over what goes on in their day-to-day practice. Agency means that one has influence over what the entire group does. Finding meaning in work is perhaps the most powerful factor in determining empathy and burnout.

The pursuit of meaning flourishes in the setting of empathy. The true practice of empathy requires continuing curiosity, as well as enough time with each patient to unleash that curiosity. As an attempt to widen the audience for this most important basic concept for patients and doctors, I had recently undertaken writing a trilogy of books using medical history as a vehicle, including <u>Savannah's Bethesda</u>. The physician energy invested in curiosity simply isn't captured by CPT codes or relative value units. Perhaps for this reason, the literature also shows that physician investment in curiosity wanes over time.

A landmark article was written by a general internist almost 25 years ago that highlights this (Fitzgerald F. Curiosity. 1999; Ann Int Med 130:70-72).

She says:

When I was a young attending at San Francisco General Hospital, morning rounds usually consisted of briefly going over the 15 to 20 patients admitted to the team the night before and then concentrating on the "interesting" ones. I was righteous and was determined to teach the house staff that there were no uninteresting patients, so I asked the resident to pick the dullest. He chose an old woman admitted out of compassion because she had been evicted from her apartment and had nowhere else to go. She had no real medical history but was simply suffering from the depredations of antiquity and abandonment. I led the protesting group of house staff to her bedside. She was monosyllabic in her responses and gave a history of no substantive content. Nothing, it seemed, had ever really happened to her. She had lived a singularly unexciting life as a hotel maid. She could not even (or would not) tell stories of famous people caught in her hotel in awkward situations. I was getting desperate; it did seem that this woman was truly uninteresting.

Finally, I asked her how long she had lived in San Francisco. "Years and years," she said was she here for the earthquake? No, she came after.

Where did she come from? Ireland. When did she come? 1912.

Had she ever been to a hospital before? Once.

How did that happen? Well, she had broken her arm. How had she broken her arm? A trunk fell on it.

A trunk? Yes. What kind of trunk? A steamer trunk.

How did that happen? The boat lurched. The boat? The boat that was carrying her to America.

Why did the boat lurch? It hit the iceberg.

Oh! What was the name of the boat? The Titanic.

She had been a steerage passenger on the Titanic when it hit the iceberg. She was injured, made it to the lifeboats, and was taken to a clinic on landing, where her broken arm was set. She now was no longer boring and immediately became an object of immense interest to the local newspapers and television stations – and the house staff.

I closed this brief reflection by saying that as we get back to in-person human contact, hopefully soon without masks, my hope for us all is that we can rekindle our curiosity and find meaning in our work.

A CONVERSATION
LINDSAY TUCKER (CRS JULY 2021)

She had hot flashes, shortness of breath, and fatigue;

Living uncomfortably every day.

There is no obvious explanation, other than weight.

However, we listened to every concern and complaint

Before having the tough conversation.

Rejection came first, then compromise, then a plan.

It's funny how some physicians still talk at people,

Rather than with them.

EVERYTHING IS FINE FOR TODAY
SHAINA MAGNESS (CRS JULY 2021)

She was a perfectly healthy forty-year-old until she felt it,

A lump which led to a lumpectomy.

Now she asks about something else she feels.

So, the doctor probes around the implant until she finds it, scar tissue, safe.

Delayed tests mean she still does not know her danger.

Genetic predisposition to one, could mean to many.

The doctor reassures that at least for today, everything is fine.

THE LONG HAUL
COLLIN MCGLONE (CRS JULY 2022)

She had quit taking her prescribed supplements,

And switched to prenatal vitamins instead.

The doctor was firm: She needed to continue taking the prescriptions.

And restart the Coumadin tomorrow night.

She was only 25, but the saddle embolus nearly took her life already.

"She will be on this medicine for the rest of her life"

HEALTH LITERACY AS AN EMPATHETIC EXERCISE
MEGAN SETTLE (MS 3 JUNE 2012)

I feel as though I have been very fortunate when it comes to exposure to health literacy education. Before I started my Family Medicine clerkship, I was exposed to health literacy discrepancies through summer programs with Trover Foundation and working in 2 different community clinics. Through these experiences I learned, among other things, that all materials given to patients should be at or below a sixth-grade reading level and I was even able to create patient handouts for a variety of topics of safety. Working to create handouts that all could understand really allowed me to grasp the disparity that can be between physician and patient communication.

Through these previous experiences and my Family Medicine clerkship, I have learned that there are many people without health literacy "hiding". Finding these hiding patients is vital to their proper health management because they will pretend they are following medical instructions as long as they possibly can. Some of the advantages of the teach back method are found when used with these hiding patients, such as helping to pin point hiding patients and then most effectively educate these patients. I have most used this technique in the community clinic in Western KY. I believe that this is because, at the community clinic, students are able to feel like patients are their own patients and feel more able to work as partners with patients toward goals in their health care. When working with preceptors, the ultimate plan for the patient is not chosen by the student so it is difficult to use or practice using the teach back method. Another aspect of the teach back method that I find challenging is using an opening so the patient does not feel inferior. At this point, the opening is challenging because it seems like acting or fake; but I do realize its importance to help the patient feel like he or she has permission to state that he or she does not understand. With practice I believe that I can move past this feeling of acting for the benefit of the patient both in the moment and for the overall improvement in health management.

Health literacy is a topic that is mistakenly overlooked by many and I think it's great that our Family Medicine program sees its importance. Unless medical students are taught that as many as 1/3 of patients do not have good health literacy, many patients would not receive the care they need due to a lack of understanding and a physician that does not perceive this or even know to look for it. Hopefully there will be many patients with better care in the future because they were taught about health literacy discrepancies and then also taught tools to work toward better health literacy.

DO YOU THINK IT WILL EVER GET BETTER? HANNAH BENNETT (MS 3 SEPTEMBER 2016)

Psychiatry is one rotation during third year where interesting patients are not in short supply. Day in and day out, I was encountering patients with a broad spectrum of mood, psychotic and personality disorders who were gracious enough to share their stories with me. One woman, in particular, made an impact on me. Laura (not her real name) is a 33-year-old mother of two boys and has been married to her husband for over ten years. She was a new patient to the psychiatrist's office where I was rotating, so I interviewed her with the attending in the room. Her story of depression, feeling hopeless, feeling like a failure and feeling overwhelmed was not particularly unique. I had seen many people with depression over the course of my rotation, and she was no different (on paper or patient logs, at least). At the end of every encounter with a patient, the psychiatrist I was working with always asked the patient if they had any questions for me- 99% of the time the patients either didn't have a question or very sweetly asked me what field I will be going into or if I enjoy medical school. However, Laura did have a question for me. She looked at me with mascara running down her face, after crying through most of our interview, and asked, "Do you think I will ever get better? Do you think there's hope for me?" With those questions, Laura, to me, epitomized and verbalized what was at the root of many patients I had encountered: the fear of never attaining relief from their mental illness.

Like many patients I had seen over the past five weeks, Laura was at the psychiatrist's office after trying, and subsequently failing, many medicines prescribed by many providers over the course of many years. But for some reason, until she posed to me the questions "Do you think I will ever get better? Do you think there's hope for me?" it hadn't occurred to me how eager these patients are for relief from their illness. It was then that I realized that her questions were echoed in all the patients I saw during this rotation: the mother with PTSD after being raped, the father who lost his life savings before seeking treatment for his alcoholism, the mother with schizophrenia who is trying her hardest to keep her mental illness from affecting her teenage son, and the grandfather with dementia and depression who is struggling to cope with his recent diagnosis of cancer.

Laura's questions really were profound for me to hear and reflect upon. I thought about the frustration she, and the other patients, must feel about not understanding why she feels this way, the defeat she feels about not having had an effective treatment thus far, and the fear she has about never feeling any different than she does now, and never getting the relief she so desperately wants, and deserves. It also gave me such an overwhelming appreciation for the psychiatrist I was working with, and how much he empowers many of his patients not just to feel better, but also to regain their lives and the part of themselves that they lost.

So, when I answered Laura, it was with a resounding, "Yes, you will get better, and you will not always feel this way. And yes, there is most certainly hope for you."

WRITTEN BY MOONLIGHT
NIKKI HARNAGE (CRS JULY 2022)

I asked, "Why are you here?"

He read to me from a notebook.

He shared a page from his past and many about his future.

Often, he spoke of the moon lighting his darkest moments.

A mistake wouldn't slow his dreams.

Tonight, I looked up to a full moon.

I imagine he saw it, too.

SHE SMILED
NIKKI HARNAGE (CRS JULY 2022)

She smiled when we pushed open the door.

She said she was good.

She wore a deep pink shirt that proclaimed she was strong.

She pulled the collar aside to show me what the surgeon did.

She smiled as we reached for the door.

Didn't she realize she had cancer?

I smiled: she was strong.

LET ME TALK
BRAD COLLINS (MS 3 MARCH 2006)

I'm the kind of person who comes in the house and puts his feet up. I make myself at home and get comfortable. I approach most situations and environments the same way, and the Hopkins County Community Clinic (HCCC) was no different. I moved to Madisonville just after taking finals at the end of second year and immediately began volunteering at the HCCC. My classmates asked me repeatedly why I was going to this clinic while studying for boards, and of course, I had a somewhat academic and rational explanation to share. Each time someone asked, I replied, "I see the free clinic as a means to gain clinical experience and integrate basic science knowledge," but to tell truth, I just wanted to talk. I craved human interaction especially after spending hours poring over review books and Q-Bank questions each day, but I found something exciting at the free clinic. I found physicians eager to quiz me with questions regarding the basic sciences, and a community that made me feel welcome in my new home.

It seems odd to me that students and residents alike now expect the weekly fellowship that clinic night now offers, but we have developed a camaraderie that far exceeds a simple weeknight search for half-priced appetizers when clinic is finished. Together, we have developed a family of sorts that attends movies, slips out of town for an occasional day trip, and hosts the sporadic cook out when the weather is nice.

Over the course of the past 14 months, I have had the opportunity to experience the continuity of care that the Trover Campus and HCCC offers University of Louisville medical students. I have come into contact with my HCCC patients in the hospital as they visit their parents following surgery and when they visit labor & delivery to hold a new grandchild. On one occasion during pediatrics, I came across Mary and her daughter Emily (not their real names). Mary was visibly nervous as the pediatric cardiologist entered the room, discarded all introductions, and barraged her with questions as to why Emily needed to see him. In fact, she was so nervous that she was unable to answer the physician's questions regarding family history and so on. Having seen Mary and her husband at the HCCC, I was well equipped to answer the physician's questions until she could gather her thoughts. As one might guess, the pediatric cardiologist was amazed when I began spouting family and social histories, but I was taken aback at the end of the visit when Mary asked me to stay behind to talk with her. She had felt very uncomfortable asking the physician questions and had refrained from doing so. Instead, Mary asked me all her questions regarding Emily's heart problems because she "trusted" me and "knew I would take the time to explain things" to her. I was floored! In that moment, I realized the unique opportunity I had simply by being involved with the HCCC. I got to see these patients in the clinic, but I also got to participate in the care of their families as a student on my various rotations.

The Hopkins County Community Clinic has nurtured me during my time in Madisonville. It has provided me fellowship with colleagues and a circle of friends while cultivating, in me, a sincere desire to play an active role in my community. I have had the opportunity to continue involvement in the clinic for over a year as a volunteer, student director, and member of the Board of Directors, and I never tire of it. I enjoy the sense of purpose I have developed in regard to the clinic and hope that my next year will be just as fruitful and exciting as the last.

MY DOCTOR ISN'T IN CONTROL OF MY HEALTH
HANNAH MARSHALL (CRS JULY 2020)

Jack (not his real name) is a patient being seen by Dr. A for a follow up appointment regarding his hypertension and lab work. He has been seeing Dr. A since the early 2000's and has developed a clear professional relationship. Jack seems to be in perfect health, slim and fit, other than his hypertension and is clearly proud of his health. He seems pleasant and tells Dr. A that he feels better than he has in years. The interaction was sufficiently short due to the lack of patient complaints.

Jack worked for a Western Kentucky school system for fourteen years as a custodian. He was never married and never had kids, but states that he currently lives with a lifelong partner that "keeps him sufficient company to not get too lonely". Jack is well dressed for his appointment and tells me that he walked to the doctor's office today out of choice. He used to run nine miles daily while he was younger and seemed to have a serious workout regimen; however, with age he now choses to walk everywhere he can rather than driving. I found this interesting considering he has a car and the heat outside, but Jack seemed very proud of the fact that he could still walk most places and get his daily exercise in.

It's evident when looking at Jack that he is thin and overall fit. He boasts constantly about his weight and activity level for his age and tells me how important it is for me to monitor my weight and try to exercise as much as possible. Jack explains to me how many years working with Dr. A he has come to learn the importance of his health, and the importance of being in control of his health. He stated that the relationship he has created with Dr. A over the years has led him to realize that he is in charge of his health rather than the doctor. It is evident through their interaction that he respects Dr. A and Dr. A respects him and his choices he has made for himself.

Jack was hesitant to talk much about himself, in true character according to Dr. A, and was more interested in my life and my school up to this point. Jack, to me, represents the true gem of healthcare: a perfect patient who prioritizes their health and life choices above anything else. On top of this, he is generally a very kind gentleman, offering his seat to me multiple times over our conversation. Jack is proud that he has never smoked, rarely drank, and most importantly never dabbled in drugs. His life choices have clearly benefitted his health as well as his mental well-being.

When talking to Jack and watching his interaction with Dr. A, I couldn't help but want to sit and talk to him for hours. Although he didn't have the most interesting and intriguing life story to tell me, he represented the reason why I want to go into healthcare. Jack represents the type of patient I want to connect with, and it is clear that his relationship with Dr. A has led him to completely prioritize his health and mental wellbeing. The impact Dr. A has made on his life has led him to a much more pleasant, healthy life whereas other patients we saw were filled with complaints that were rooted in years of bad habits and unhealthy choices.

I have never met a patient like Jack who is such a caring individual who radiates within himself and within others.

When I asked Jack if he had any advice for me as a future physician, he simply stated that, "You need to remain healthy. Practice what you preach and always care for others the way you would want to be cared for. You will make it far with that attitude."

PATIENCE FOR PATIENTS
AMBER SHADOAN (MS 3 MARCH 2018)

It was an average day on the behavioral health unit. As a medical student, morning pre-rounding consists of seeing the patients newly admitted since the previous day, and reporting back to the attending. H was an 83-year-old man who presented to the hospital overnight from a nursing home with acutely altered mental status including outbursts of agitation and unusual behavior. After being treated medically for pneumonia, his mental status had still not improved so he was admitted to the behavioral health unit.

On interviewing H, he was a very pleasant man with an old-fashioned cordiality. He appeared tired and stated that he did not feel well. I could tell it took a great deal of effort for him to speak and he quickly drifted off into talking about getting into his fishing boat so that we could catch some fish. Dr. A was the attending psychiatrist on the unit and began rounds with H. He was aghast at the long medication list, and was immediately suspicious that it could be a source of the mental status changes. After speaking with H, Dr. A put in orders to decrease the dosage of opiate pain medication and discontinue some others that may not be necessary, such as those for acid reflux and allergy medications. After that, it was a waiting game. Each day Dr. A took report from the night-shift nursing staff on H' behavior, and continued to slowly adjust his medications with a goal of prescribing the minimum number of medications that are necessary. Over time he gradually stopped having agitated behaviors and was able to sleep through the night. During morning rounds, H steadily appeared stronger and more alert. When he was finally ready to be discharged, we had a family meeting with his two sons and daughter in law. They expressed amazement and gratitude to Dr. A for the changes they have seen in their father. They stated that his mental status is better now than it has been for months. Over the past year, as they described, his cognition had steadily declined until he was groggy during the day and mostly unable to interact with family, then agitated and behaving badly at night-time. They felt like a part of their father had been returned to them at a time when they thought it was gone forever.

The family meeting had a great impact on me as a medical student who is interested in geriatric care. I feel that too frequently we observe patients with unnecessarily long medication lists with a "that's a shame" attitude, and not with an attitude of looking for change or improvement. I saw a man enter the hospital as someone who could easily be dismissed as demented and then later discharged with a level of clarity he hadn't experienced in months. It was such an incredible moment to witness his children's tears of joy as they thanked the doctor for giving them more time with the father they had always known.

As a future physician, I learned a great lesson from H. I will be more cautious and more exhaustive in my search to find alternative causes for an elderly patient's declining mental status before labeling it as something irreparable. I will not passively accept a dreadfully long medication list and think of it as a shame. I will do what I can to decrease it and try to find ways to improve my patient's quality of life in doing so. I will especially be cautious in assigning new medications with a newfound awareness that each new drug comes with potential consequences that should be weighed carefully against consequences and re-assessed periodically. I hope to see more cases like H and never be too quick in judgement.

RHYTHM, NOT THE BLUES
LEEANDRA CLEAVER (MS 3 OCTOBER 2020)

The phrase "rhythm and blues" always reminds me of the deep, soulful music of the past. Music has the ability to transport people to their most safe, but also sometimes their most vulnerable, places. The genre of music one enjoys really does say something about who they are. I recently had a patient who exemplified this completely, and I will never forget my time with him.

I met Mr. L on the second week of my psychiatry clerkship. I had spent the first week of the clerkship observing and learning from those around me, trying to absorb as much as I possibly could. By the second week, I knew that I would be on my own to interview patients. I walked in that Monday morning ready to work with the new patients on the adult wing. As I opened the doors to the unit, I happened upon my attending in the Geriatric hallway, conversing with a man in his 60s. The man was clinging to a walker for support, clearly confused, and somewhat agitated. He was demanding to know the reason as to why he was in the hospital and was describing how he had every capability of taking care of himself. By the expressions on both of their faces, I could tell that the conversation was not productive, and that Mr. L was growing increasingly upset. My attending was trying to calm him and explain to him that he was safe in the hospital, but to no avail. Eventually, he led Mr. L over to a seat by the television and told him he would speak with him later. By this point, I had wandered over, clearly trying to figure out why this man was so upset. The curious medical student in me was enthralled by the interaction. My attending then suggested that I go sit with him and see if I could figure out what was going on. We made plans to meet later to talk about the patient, his diagnosis, and the plan moving forward.

As soon as I sat down next to Mr. L, his sharp brown eyes latched on to mine and he said, "Wow girl, you have some curly hair!" My first reaction was pure shock, and then laughter by how abrupt and how different his affect was from just a few minutes prior. He then laughed boisterously alerting the nurses and the social worker nearby. By this point, his aggressiveness had melted as he started telling me his story. He was a musician, which I immediately related to since I also grew up listening to all sorts of music. He was a member of a jazz band and knew how to "tickle the ivories." Others were asking him questions about the songs he played: his repeated response was "I play only smooth jazz. You don't really play specific songs." When I added, "Right? Isn't jazz about improv? You play what you feel," he knew he had a friend in me. We talked more about his time of playing music in Detroit, his love of Motown and Michael Jackson, and the many instruments he knew how to play. He then told me about his time as a pilot in the Marine Corps, his family, and where he grew up. He was a born storyteller with every piece of his puzzle reaching his eyes and smile.

I initially did not realize he had schizophrenia. It was with observing him each day that I witnessed the additive effects of his delusions, flat affect, and worsening non-compliance with medications. He became very disorganized in conversation, transitioning one minute from talking about God, to being angry with his brother, all the while inserting repeatedly and randomly that he could indeed take care of himself. One particular instance that resonated with me was when he spoke of how God was telling him that he wouldn't have to go to another institution. He said to me "Curly, God told me I'm going to get to go home today. And my oh my, he has painted me the most beautiful summer day! I've missed my summer being in here."

Mr. L recently had a court hearing regarding his inability to properly care for himself and his need to receive inpatient care. I saw the worry in his eyes, the frustration in his lack of insight, and the sheer sadness that accompanied the final decision. I will never forget the distraction that the window in our conference room provided as the judge read aloud his decision. Mr. L was instead focused on three birds that were flying outside of the window.

What Mr. L doesn't realize is that I will forever remember him. Yes, he was my first patient diagnosed with Schizophrenia that I helped care for, but I also realized that he was defined by so much more than his illness. His creativity as both a storyteller and a musician came through allowing us to form a bond. As a medical student, I have been told by numerous physicians to always look at the person behind the patient. I have heard this saying so many times, but this is one of the first times that I was able to personally make the connection. Patients have illness, but they are not defined by that said illness. Mr. L entrusted me with his story; the things he loved to do, the places he visited, and his love of music. I will take this with me in every patient encounter that I have moving forward.

Towards the beginning of his admission, our social worker brought in a keyboard for Mr. L to play. I opened the double doors onto the Behavioral Health Unit to a beautiful melody, followed by intricate runs of the keys.

I teared up as he played *Somewhere Over the Rainbow*. He then promised me that after I finished my work for the day, he would play a song especially for me. When I asked what kind of song, he replied, "I don't know, Curly. But I play the rhythm, not the blues."

THE IMPORTANCE OF MEDICAL HISTORY
MYRA IRVIN (MS 4 OCTOBER 2014)

I gained some insight about communication and continuity of care when I saw a patient being treated for schizophrenia. The patient's antipsychotic medications had quieted the voices she had been hearing for years, and allowed her to live a normal life. She was a widowed lady who lived alone in an apartment complex. As the follow up visit continued, the patient explained that she had recently seen a new doctor and had been diagnosed with Parkinson's disease.

She did not appear overly concerned with her new diagnosis, and pulled out a crumbled piece of paper with a long list of drug names. The doctor who had diagnosed her with Parkinson's disease had prescribed several new medications. When she filled them about a week ago, her bill was over $800, and she appeared to be distraught by this amount. She was sincere in her efforts to comply with the doctor's orders and scraped up enough money to pay for the first month's prescription. However, she expressed deep concern that she would be unable to afford these medications long term.

When we saw the medication list, we immediately saw a potential problem. She was being treated with the standard medications that one would expect with the diagnoses of Parkinson's disease. However, she was also being treated with medications with similar effects from us for her residual schizophrenia. It quickly became evident to us that her medications were counteracting each other.

Our patient had put full trust in her physicians to provide the best care. She was only worried that she would not be able to afford their recommendations. We changed dosages and removed a few medications to come to a better balance that should help with the Parkinson's symptoms and still suppress the voices. I was frustrated and upset because she had spent $800 of her limited income to get her first month's prescriptions of medications that she may not need.

When questioned further, she admitted that she had not revealed her schizophrenia treatment to this other physician. She conceded that she perceived psychiatric illness and medical disease as separate entities. Sadness filled my heart as I realized that this one step in miscommunication was potentially causing these problems.

Most of my frustration was because the doctor who diagnosed and treated her Parkinson's disease had failed to gather a thorough history. Although she admitted to being less than forthcoming with this physician, it is still the responsibility of the health care provider to create an environment that allows gathering of a complete history. This showed a lack of communication between physician and patient as well as between providers.

What was also disquieting to me was the issue of prescribing expensive medications to patients who can't afford them. The reality is that most patients are on a budget. The physician who prescribed the Parkinson's medications neglected to inquire about costs to the patient. From this experience I learned several important lessons that I want to carry into my practice. When a patient presents with a new onset of symptoms, it is imperative that a physician collect a thorough history. It is also vital that a physician address how a patient will pay for the medications, tests, or procedures that are ordered. If a physician does not take the time to address this issue, it is likely that a patient will be unable to complete treatment. Failure of patient compliance is not always due to uncooperative patients. As a result of this patient encounter, I plan on making it habit to discuss access and cost of treatments and medications I order."

THE PATIENT WITH NINE LIVES
TIFFANY SIMPSON (MS 3 SEPTEMBER 2010)

I would like to preface this with the fact that I love old people. They have such special stories to tell about a time that is far gone: a time that I realize included hard work but created individuals that were resilient and didn't take for granted the fruits of their labors. It seems in my generation we have been handed all too much and have grown to expect certain things and never learn to appreciate them. In Mr. C it was his resiliency against all odds that amazed me and his eagerness to return home to his family and most importantly his dog that left a lasting impression.

Mr. C was a 77-year-old that I met in the Critical Care Unit on the first day of IM on my Cardiology rotation. He was sitting up in bed eating his eggs from breakfast. I knocked on the door and introduced myself and he stopped eating, pushed his tray aside, adjusted what was left of the hair on his head, and gave me a huge grin and a joyful good morning. Mr. C was very sick and had a long list of "working diagnoses" on the computer and many medicines that I combed through daily. Despite his illness, every day that week was the same grin and good morning and maybe a story or two about his family and dog that he was so ready to return home to and see. His wife would call the nurse every day and make sure he ate his lunch because, as you know, eating everything on your plate makes you better, or at least she was convinced of that.

Over the weekend Mr. C had a stroke which left him intubated and paralyzed on the right side. It was really sad to go in and not see his bright and hopeful smile. I moved on to a new rotation but would occasionally check in to see how he was doing. In a few days his condition improved and he was taken off the ventilator. During the next month he continued to fight despite many episodes of minor CVAs, MIs, and scary flash pulmonary edema. It was like taking one step forward one day and three steps back the next. Mr. C became a patient of the hospitalists whose service I was now on. I never got assigned Mr. C but we met every morning so I was updated on his condition daily. I knew Mr. C would not make it back home, but I had tremendous respect for the man that I met, although there really wasn't much left of that man who was now laying hopeless in his bed. My peers didn't get the chance of meeting Mr. C when he was somewhat himself and only spoke of him as "the patient with nine lives." The hospitalists worked hard to make Mr. C's family understand his grave condition and to make him a DNR. It had come to a point where science and medicine had retrieved Mr. C from death so many times it had become cruel, each painful time only bringing back a smaller and smaller percentage of the person I had met that first day. Mr. C passed away last

Friday and even though he wasn't returning to the home he worked for, I like to think he finally got rest in another home that he deserved.

This patient was such a memorable patient for me because with him I had many firsts. He was my first patient, my first critical care patient, and first patient where I witnessed the dying process. Mr. C was a special person to me and what I took most from the whole experience was that not everyone feels the same way about their patients. I understand Mr. C was a complicated patient but there were so many unkind things said about the situation. In the restroom today there was a sign that said, "Be Kind---you are taking care of someone's brother, sister, mother, father, grandparent." I just thought that was so fitting for this reflection paper because I think many people forgot that there was a person laying in there that was important to so many others and many took those special relationships for granted. It was sad to see us painfully prolonging his life but his family was waiting for a miracle and that should have been respected instead of being turned into a joke. The fact that he was such a fighter should have been admired rather than disregarded.

I think this experience will make me not just a better physician but a better person. It will be a reminder to me to be more cautious of how my words can affect others whether in the hospital, at work, or with my family and friends. I'm sure there will be many frustrating situations in my future and I hope I always give my patients the respect that I would want for my own family members.

-- "Be completely humble and gentle; be patient, bearing with one another in love" -- Ephesians 4:2

YOU DID WHAT?
SARAH FISHER (MS 4 OCTOBER 2014)

My patients have taught me about accepting others exactly how they are. This lesson has been explored extensively with my continuity patients at the free clinic in Madisonville, staffed by the Trover Rural Track medical students. I have patients who continue to smoke despite counseling, patients who take their medications the way they want to take them, and patients who hate the idea of needles despite their HbA1c of 10.1. At first, I was frustrated; I couldn't understand why my patients didn't want to help themselves. Rather than resenting them, I dedicated myself to understanding my patients better. My patient who would not stop smoking? She was nervous, and has cut down with the help of an anti-depressant to control her anxiety. My patient who didn't take her medication consistently? She was overwhelmed by the sheer number of medications and wanted a consistent provider. The diabetic who refused insulin? He thought it would make his diabetes worse because his dad's diabetes continued to progress after starting insulin. Once I understood my patients and accepted where they were at rather than where I wanted them to be, I was able to take better care of them.

My continuity patients have also taught me about celebrating every victory, no matter how small. I never thought that I would celebrate a patient knowing the name of a medication, or bringing a log of blood sugars. Little did I know that I would be relishing and glowing with pride for my patients for these accomplishments. I have high-fived my patients for losing 5 pounds, increasing their breaths on the incentive spirometer, and even increasing their exercise to walking around the block once a day. This same pride translated to my home life. I celebrate every victory of my family and friends, cheering them on in every facet. Whether it is passing an important exam or finding the perfect dress, every milestone should be enjoyed.

GASTRIC STIMULATOR MISHAP
TATE BURRIS (CRS JULY 2020)

Mrs. W is a 48-year-old woman who has spent the majority of her life in Western Kentucky with her mom dad and two older brothers. Her family moved to Oklahoma for two years when she was growing up, but quickly returned because they missed being close to their family. Family is very important to Mrs. W. She has been married to her husband for 5 years. She has four kids as well as four grandkids who all live relatively close and they continue to maintain a very close relationship. When asked, "What is the most important thing to her in your life?" she says her children and her grandchildren. Mrs. W is no stranger to the medical field as she has some training in being a medical assistant until she decided to focus on taking care of her house and kids as a stay-at-home mom.

Mrs. W is also no stranger to being a patient in the medical field as she has struggled with gastroparesis for the past 23 years. She said she has constantly been in and out of doctors' offices for her entire life and sadly they have not always been positive encounters. A few months ago, she was struggling with some very intense pain in her stomach. She didn't think too much about it at first as she has dealt with gastroparesis for a long time. The pain continued to worsen and she finally decided to go to the emergency room. While there she said that she waited for what seemed like hours all for the doctors to tell her that there was nothing wrong with her and sent her on her way. The pain continued to grow so she decided to go to the emergency room in Madisonville for a second opinion. While there, the doctors realized that a gastric stimulator that she had was malfunctioning and giving her problems. They immediately rushed her back for emergency surgery where they removed the stimulator. She claims that she is feeling much better since the procedure but that she was confused as to why the doctors in the other town had missed it. She said that she felt as if the other doctors didn't care and just wanted to get her out as soon as possible.

In reflecting over Mrs. W's story, I was touched by how much she cared for and loved her family. This touched me because family has always been important to me and it seems like in today's day and age, I have seen so many people grow away from their family that it was wonderful to see this woman whose whole life has been so family oriented. And as touching as that is, it also pained me to hear her say that she felt like some of the doctors she had seen didn't really care about her, and just wanted to get her gone as quick as possible. As physicians, it is our job to take care of our patients because we genuinely care about the well-being of our patients. Just the way she sounded when talking about this made it obvious that she was really upset by those doctors. This really reiterated just how important it is for physicians to genuinely care about our patients and take their time with them so they can be fully engaged and do the best job they possibly can.

A CHANCE FOR A FRESH START
BLAKE EDMONSON (PRE-MATRIC JUNE 2020)

Mrs. K is from Western Kentucky. She has one daughter who she adores dearly and wants the best. Her daughter is fourteen years old and going through a tough time at home with the "quarantine" situation. However, they plan to make some big changes this summer that will definitely add some excitement to their lives. Mrs. K and her daughter love to fish and spend time together outside. She recalls that fishing was her favorite family bonding experience growing up as a child in Central Kentucky. Her parents are separated, and both live nearby in the state. She said they haven't always had the best relationships, but she tries to keep in contact frequently throughout each month. The separation of her parents while she was in high school was tough on the family. This drove her to move out after high school graduation and seek a new life with a different purpose.

Upon graduating from high school, she attended a local community college for about a year before entering directly into the work force. She worked in many different fields of business and gained many experiences that made her into a well-rounded employee. The majority of her employments were in the food industry where she has acquired "countless stories" of funny or wild experiences on the job. She married young at the age of twenty-two to a man she had met through one of her previous jobs. He was a sweet man to her at first, but later became very controlling of her and her daughter.

Mrs. K has since had a hard time, mentally and physically. She recalls many times where her husband has been very demanding and obsessive over her "whereabouts" and "what she had been up to". The toll of this on top of many other incidents has led her to seek help medically. She has been on anxiety and depression medications and has finally found the right combination that does not have side effects that are worse than the initial symptoms. She said many of the medications she tried helped with the anxiety and depression but gave her very vivid and lucid nightmares, many that were too intense to even discuss. However, the new medications have allowed her to feel better overall and even sleep soundly without lucid dreams.

In the next month, her divorce from her husband will be official, and she plans to pack up and move to Florida with her fourteen-year-old daughter. There she will seek out a fresh start and better living conditions. She is excited about this new phase of life and wants the best for her daughter. The idea of a complete change of scenery was scary to her at first, but she is more excited about the idea of new chapter of life for her daughter and herself.

BABIES ARE LIKE A REAL SPECIAL PET
JORDAN HARBIN (CRS JULY 2022)

Babies are easy.

Like a really special pet that you feed, nurture, protect

Children though, children like to pretend

They want to play games, socialize.

They make me feel foolish.

Somehow, they do

Siblings make it hard to hear

Heart sounds, parents, your thoughts.

They don't listen.

I just want to hold all the babies.

THESE PEOPLE NEED US
JORDAN HARBIN (CRS JULY 2021)

The first two patients had Great Smoky Mountains t-shirts,

They reminded me of a trip with my family.

I thought about their own families, waiting to hear about their doctor's appointment.

Or maybe they didn't care. Maybe they were alone.

This isn't the fast-paced environment of my younger days.

But these people need us.

BASKET CASE
ALEXIS HEAD (PRE-MATRIC JUNE 2023)

I had the opportunity to interview Ms. K on the inpatient Psychiatry unit. She is a 19-year-old that identifies as a female and is originally from Madisonville. The patient lives with nine siblings and a mother. Before admission, the patient worked three jobs. Ms. K explained that high anxiety and insecurity cause stress in her life. The patient mentioned that being around others usually exacerbates that insecurity.

Ms. K worked three jobs as a distraction from these thoughts and anxieties. The patient had recently lost her dad in a car accident. This death has caused the patient to fear death and the death of other family members. Ms. K explained that oftentimes a visualization of her death would appear in her head. This same visualization occurs regarding her mother's life. However, Ms. K's mother mentally abuses her and calls the patient a "basket case" regularly. This mental abuse caused Ms. K to pursue a relationship with a male. The patient explained that the boyfriend was "narcissistic and verbally abusive."

This was the second time that Ms. K had been admitted here. The first time, the patient came on their own accord due to "feeling down" and self-described manic episodes. This first visit ended in discharge a few days after admission. This second admission was requested by Ms. K as well. The patient had an incident with her boyfriend. Ms. K was in the car with her boyfriend when he made a few remarks to her. Ms. K asked him to stop the car and Ms. K pulled him out of the car and "beat him up." The patient hit him because "he's a guy and couldn't hit me back." She ran away from the incident and requested admission. Ms. K expected to be discharged the day after this interview. The patient said that the group sessions and isolation from family have improved her overall mental health.

The interview was conducted in Ms. K's room around 3 pm. The patient was laying down with the lights off before the interview.

RELIGIOUS FREEDOM
HOPE DULL-POTTER (PRE-MATRIC JUNE 2023)

She was sitting in the main open sitting area for patients on the inpatient Psychiatry unit. She was a girl not much younger than myself. It was her long, braided pigtails and friendly disposition that caught my attention. As I got closer to the table, she got up to move. I said, "Hi, I'm going to be a medical student this fall and was wondering if I could ask you a few questions about yourself that will help me become a better physician one day?" She happily obliged and we started walking towards her room. This is where I learned her story: the story of Miss "E".

Miss "E" was the youngest of three children. From an early age, she observed the actions and mistakes of her older siblings which gave her a desire to achieve in all areas of life. Her earliest memory as a child was her grandma grasping her and warmly saying, "You're my perfect little angel." The feeling of having to be perfect loomed over Miss "E" like a dark cloud. No matter how many awards and scholarships were allotted, she knew perfect was unattainable for any human. Miss "E" finds refuge in her faith as a devoted Christian, often recounting scriptures by memory throughout the interview. She stated this was the sixth place she had been admitted, but the only one which allowed her to partake in religious freedom. For the first time in a long time, she felt confident again. This newfound confidence has given her a voice, and one she wants healthcare professionals to hear in order to deliver better care to the patients they serve.

Determinedly, Miss "E" points out that her goal is not to be on medication for the rest of her life. The idea of her senses being dulled to the voice of the Holy Spirit was not only unattractive, but not an option for how she wants to live her life. Miss "E" states the doctor-to-doctor communication may be a form of the classic game of telephone, often feeling like what she relays to one doctor may not be what it sounded like to the original ears. She recounts the beginnings of mistrust in people starting with her parent's divorce. Then, when admission length and additional criteria were being given by physicians, the mistrust began again. With a genuine desire to see change, Miss "E" gives two pieces of advice that align with her values. The first being, "We cannot neglect the soul.

Equally important are the mind, body, and spirit.". Secondly, "A place to sing outside instead of isolation. Singing soothes the soul." Her ultimate dream is to marry her boyfriend and travel to every continent, sharing the gospel with those around her. Miss "E" is a capable young woman who will achieve whatever she sets her mind to.

ROCK AND A HARD PLACE
LAUREN TROUT (PRE-MATRIC JUNE 2023)

"I was born 28 years ago." Not long after his birth, the patient's dad was arrested. Then when he was two years old, his parents got divorced. He grew up on a small farm in Eastern Kentucky with several great danes and beagles and a few other small farm animals, but no siblings. He loved being around all the animals and said those were some of his best child-hood memories. He played basketball for most of his life and even won two state championships off his free throws.

After graduating high school, he attended Murray State University major-ing in psychology with a minor in biology. He went into this with the in-tention of pursuing a career at a behavioral health facility. Unfortunately, he only attended MSU for a year before transferring to a vocational school because he started partying too much and got involved in some bad things, which he didn't specify. This may play a role in the court-ordered admission from a local group home.

The patient really likes being outside and partaking in several outdoor activities. He enjoys going for walks, going to the park, going fishing, and occasionally playing basketball still. While he doesn't have a family of his own yet, he mentioned that he would eventually like to and if he had a son, he would get him involved with baseball since it is much less grueling than basketball.

He related his life to the song *Rock and a Hard Place* by Bailey Zimmerman, but not in the relationship sense that most people would infer the song to mean. He meant it more in the sense that his life hasn't been easy, and it has led him to be put in a place where it literally feels like he is just stuck between a rock and a hard place. The patient says he feels like he is doing better, and his dad and paternal grandparents have been his biggest motivation in getting better and turning his life around. He calls them often and they try to keep him positive and keep him on the right track.

When he gets out, he plans to go back to his hometown where he'd be closer to his family and get a job. He mentioned a job driving a forklift that he had before he was admitted. He has high hopes for his mental health after leaving the facility and seems to have a steady support system to keep him on the right track. He plans to get back into playing basketball for fun in the future and create a steady life for himself.

WORKING ON MY ATTITUDE
JORDAN HARBIN (PRE-MATRIC JUNE 2023)

Ms. B had a great childhood. She grew up in a house with her father, mother, brother, and sister. She was the youngest. She said her dad always wanted to be a pediatrician, and growing up it was like having a pediatrician in the house all the time. She often cleaned her neighbors in- ground pool, and in exchange was allowed to spend many summer days swimming. One of her favorite childhood memories was having her friends over to camp in tents in her backyard.

She graduated high school and attended some college before working as a secretary and a nurse aid. She enjoyed her interactions with people, but always wanted to be in legal administration. She was 4 courses shy of completing her college degree, something she plans to do in the future. At some point in time her loving father changed, becoming mean and uncaring. She says he only liked kids, not teenagers and adults, and when she and her siblings grew up their father stopped treating them well. Part of the reason she was unable to finish her degree was because he controlled her finances. Her boyfriend at the time helped her sue someone and was awarded a million dollars, but her father never let her have the money. After he changed, she states that he was mean for the rest of his life.

For fun she enjoys watching football and basketball with her friends. She also really likes to shop, go on walks, and decorate her house. Her ideal future involves her owning a home with a fence, getting married, adopting some kids, and getting a big dog. Her favorite dogs are collies, like Lassie.

Her biggest health concern is working on her attitude. She feels that she gets stuck in cycles of thinking about the worst possible outcomes, and needs to focus on thinking more positively and trusting what her doctors say. Her main fear is that she is going to fall, possible break a hip, and lose her ability to walk. She is greatly concerned about maintaining her ability to walk. Talking about her fears helps, and hearing the doctors say she is doing good is encouraging. She constantly reminds herself to look on the bright side, and hopes to live on her own when she leaves.

Exacerbation of these negative feelings led Ms. B to seek emergency care. Feelings of anxiety became overwhelming, and she felt the need for medical attention. Upon assessment in the emergency department, she responded positively to having thoughts of hurting herself. It was decided that the best course of action would be to admit her to the hospital for monitoring and treatment until her condition resolved.

Ms. B was an extremely pleasant person to talk to and had an interesting story to tell. Even though her main complaint was a negative attitude, she was very positive when discussing her future goals and willingness to continue receiving treatment. Having no experience interviewing psychiatric patients I don't know if I did a good job or not. I tried to talk as little as possible, allowing Ms. B to speak as long as she wished in response to short prompts. Verifying this information was difficult without having any prior knowledge of the patient's history or medical conditions. Much of her story seemed realistic, but some parts of her story seemed a little outlandish or hard to follow. Further exposure to this type of patient will certainly make this process more efficient.

LIFE IS A HIGHWAY
EMILY BOLINGER (PRE-MATRIC JUNE 2023)

I saw her early that morning in group therapy, snapping a rubber band against her hand, looking at a paper with suggestions for coping with stress. When asked about coping mechanisms she would try, she mumbled under her breath "playing sports".

Entering her room later, she was clearly resting but raised her head to begin telling me about her childhood in New York. She grew up playing volleyball, softball, and basketball. She came to Madisonville to stay at a rehabilitation facility. She looked no older than 25, and the complacent look on her face told me this isn't the first time she has explained herself to a doctor.

She has a twin sister and an older brother. I learned she has taken many family vacations to beaches. She likes to tan. I asked about her fresh tan, and she told me the rehabilitation center has them do a lot of outdoor activities. She detailed that this center does not really understand "people like her with schizoaffective disorders", but they try their best to accommodate. This patient was originally diagnosed with bipolar disorder 8 years ago then eventually told she was schizophrenic 3 years after that. I could tell that she has never felt like there is a place for her, like she has always been different and didn't understand why. I asked her if this diagnosis helped make sense of the things for her. She said yes.

After high school, she went to college up north. This time was cut short when her mother was diagnosed with cancer and was in a severe car accident. She had to go home and take care of her mother along with the rest of her family. After this, there are some holes in the story, but I could tell her symptoms started to lower her quality of life drastically and her family's ability to give her the care she needed. She spent some time working part time for the YMCA, but she ultimately could not live a successful life with her hallucinations and episodes of psychosis. This is what landed her in rehabilitation facilities. These specific facilities are directed towards patients with a history of substance abuse, so they do not necessarily have the resources she specifically needs. She wishes doctors would understand her and hear what she is saying. She wants a new outpatient psychiatrist.

She hears her deceased mother sometimes. She started hearing her mother ask for help, and this made her think she was still alive. This is why she was sent to the hospital. Her father will not give her the mortuary's number to ask if her mother is dead. She does not understand why. And she mentioned this multiple times.

She is a praying person. Music makes her happy. Her favorite band is Rascal Flatts, and she loves to sing to *Life is a Highway*. She hopes her dad will comes visit next month, and her life would be better if she moved to a rehabilitation center closer to her family in New York.

TO DIE FOR
JACK DODDS (CRS JULY 2023)

Most people in the hospital want to return to health so that they can return home to see their families again. This 78-year-old patient, who we will call Janice, was no different. In the hospital for heart failure and chronic COPD, Janice's goal for her care was simply to be able to get home as soon as possible to see her family. She described how often she was called by people trying to convince her to change her insurance companies. She told us she loves to respond with "I'll call the police and see if they can't put a stop to you guys always bothering me". What those insurance companies don't know is that behind the 78-year-old hospital patient, there is a lifetime of stories worth sharing that they don't even care about. Having grown up in a town of 2,000 people, faith and family were at the roots of Janice's beliefs. She grew up across the street from the church she attended with her parents. She started high school but had to drop out and work to help the family she cared so much for. She was baptized at 16 and remembers it saying "It was one of the most important days of my life".

Eventually she was able to return to high school and graduate before getting a job at a factory that she kept faithfully for 35 years. In those years, she loved to sew blue jeans and cook for her six children. She tells us that her children say that her banana pudding was "to die for". Her health started to decline when she was diagnosed with COPD, which she has now had for 15 years. In those 15 years, she has become dependent on her children and grandchildren to care for her. She can no longer do the things she once loved to do. No more sewing blue jeans and no more banana pudding. After checking into the hospital for shortness of breath, she found out that her heart was failing too. This diagnosis prompted the discussion of hospice, which she didn't quite seem to understand, continuously refusing. As much as we tried to explain, she would not have it. Simply listening to this one patient made me come to several realizations. The first was that there are much worse things to be experiencing than a

Biochemistry exam. Janice's story was also a show of devotion and faith to the things she cares most about, being her family. Not able to walk and hardly able to talk, all she could think about was seeing her grandchildren again. The reason this story really hit home for me was that Janice very much reminded me of my own grandmother. We are blessed that he does not suffer from the same health conditions, but they are very much alike. This helped me reaffirm the realization that behind each patient, behind each digital chart, is a story waiting to be told.

HANGING MY BRAIN UP
RILEY ERIKSEN (PRE-CLINICAL JULY 2023)

While observing in the psychiatric unit, I had the opportunity to speak with a 70-year-old great-grandmother. She had checked herself into the unit after experiencing some episodes of psychosis. At first, I watched the medical student on rotation perform a memory test with her and then asked if I could interview her. She graciously agreed and our discussion began.

We started off talking about her childhood. She explained how she lived with her parents and siblings. Her mother worked as a housekeeper and her father worked for an oil company. Among her siblings were 3 brothers, two of whom were significantly older. She also had a sister who was 5 years younger. Unfortunately, she lost both of her parents around 10 years ago, and she is now left with only one brother who lives in California.

As she talked about her childhood, the memory that stood out was of her dog and puppies. Her dog H became a mom to 4 puppies, two of which she named after former presidents. She also recalled going fishing and hunting with her father, who would encourage her to get over her fear of taking the fish off the hooks. When it came to school, her favorite subjects were math and spelling. Of the sports at her school, she particularly enjoyed track, especially when they did the long jumps.

After high school, she married her husband at 18 and then welcomed her first daughter at 21. Though she had wanted to pursue higher education, financial issues stopped her. Her dad would not agree to submit his income information so that she could apply for financial aid, and she could not afford going without it. She explained how she tried to convince him by saying it was an investment in the family, but he still refused. Instead, she worked as a medical transcriptionist and later started school to be a physician's assistant but did not finish.

She now has 4 grandchildren, one of which recently graduated with a political science degree and graduated magna cum laude. Her other granddaughter has 2 children, and she says she loves to make art boxes for her great-grandchildren. In her leftover free time, she enjoys looking into her genealogy. So far, she has discovered that she is related to many famous people. Currently, her main goal for her health is to figure out whatever is "hanging [her] brain up." Once she does that, she would love for her future to include spending time with her grandkids and breeding dogs.

When I asked her about advice for me, she told me about watching a patient's face and body language when I talk to them, a trick she learned from her husband who played poker. She also said I should always make sure that if I am asking a patient to give me their best, I need to make sure that I am giving them mine. Talking with her reminded me of talking to my own grandmother, and making that connection really helped show me the rich lives patients lead outside of the doctor's office, as well as the important roles they serve in the lives of others. Knowing that she was someone else's grandmother gave me a new perspective of her healthcare goals and showed me another layer of the importance of caring for people.

TIME TO LISTEN
EMILY AMYX (PRE-CLINICAL JULY 2023)

The patient that I interviewed was a 40 y/o female who was from Illinois. She had come to town with her significant other for a camping trip. During this trip, she and her significant other had a falling out. She called her mother to let her know that she would be ending her life that night. In response, her mother called the local Police Department, which then took this patient to the Emergency Room to be evaluated. This is where I conducted my interview with this patient.

This patient grew up on a farm in Illinois with many pets and animals. Her favorite animals growing up were her horses. Some of her favorite childhood memories involved her spending time with her horse, going to the beach with her family, and going to pigeon forge with her family. Some of her favorite subjects in school were math and science. She didn't play any organized sports growing up but loved playing basketball and running with her friends. Additional hobbies that she enjoys now are fishing, hiking, and anything to do with the outdoors. When asked about health issues and concerns, she mentioned that money has always been an issue and being away from family was another issue. The patient explained that she is excited to go back home after her hospital stay and spend time with her family. She says that she thinks that she will feel much better once she is back home with them. When asked what her best future might look like, she said that she just wants her entire family to be happy, healthy, live well, and also get more money. Finally, when asked what advice she had for me as a future physician, she said that I just need to make sure that I listen to patients.

Overall, I really enjoyed talking to this patient about her life, her experiences, and what brought her here. She was very warm and inviting. This experience taught me to make sure to take time with patients and allow them to talk and tell their owns stories without interjecting. This allows more trust in the relationship and also helps you get to know your patient better, which you can then use to treat them better.

CHAPTER 9

55 Word Stories

"I would have written a shorter letter, but I did not have the time."

This quote is generally attributed to French philosopher and mathematician Blaise Pascal. Similar sentiments have been attributed to John Locke, Woodrow Wilson, Benjamin Franklin, and Mark Twain. Anyone who has tried to distill a powerful interaction with a patient into just a few words knows the power of reflection that is required. In our summer programs for college rural scholars and medical students, we used the style published recently (Gramelspacher and Cummins. Academic Medicine. 95 (10): 2020 p.1541) as a template. What they wrote ranged from a simple objective description to the depths of human pathos. They follow here, and I know you will appreciate them as much as I did. Bill Crump, MD.

I IGNORED YOU...
NIKKI HARNAGE (CRS JULY 2022)

Before she opened the door, the doctor leaned over: "This patient does whatever he wants."

"Do you exercise?"

"I walk to my truck and back."

"How's your diet?"

"I eat whatever I want."

"Didn't we talk about that last time... and the time before that?"

"Yeah, I ignored you."

"As long as you realize it."

PRAYING FOR PATIENT CHANGE
COLIN MCGLONE (CRS JULY 2022)

New Patient - Establishing Care

The urinalysis was positive,

For methamphetamine and THC,

But she really hasn't used it recently, she's sure.

Yes, she's aware cigarettes are unhealthy,

But she is going to stop.

Yes, she's aware that she is in the second trimester of her pregnancy,

She is trying to get things turned around.

I can only imagine what circumstances led her to this point,

And I can only pray she is serious about change, for her and her child's sake.

HOMEBOUND
LINDSAY TUCKER (CRS JULY 2021)

As soon as we walked in, I could tell she was exhausted and sick. Another covid exposure that unfortunately fell in between doses of the vaccine. However, she wasn't concerned for herself. She was worried about her homebound mother, who has been unable to receive a vaccine, not for lack of trying. I wish people didn't get left behind.

CARING
SHAINA MAGNESS (CRS JULY 2021)

A new patient, this one will take some time.

Medical History:

Congestive Heart Failure (stable, but has not seen her cardiologist in 6 months)

Chronic Pancreatitis (unknown cause)

Hepatitis A (treated, but not vaccinated)

The lists go on and on of related and unrelated conditions, medications, and allergens.

This patient has many stories to share, but most of them come back to one thing:

"For the past two years my husband is very sick and being treated in Louisville, so I just have not had the time to take care of myself."

"Well, you know you need to take care of yourself, so you can keep supporting him, so here is what we are going to do…"

PATIENT AND FRIEND
NIKKI HARNAGE (CRS JULY 2021)

Patient and friend.

"Doc, I know this is the end."

18, 12, 6, hours to live.

"What am I supposed to do?"

I want pray,

but he offers all he can give:

"It's up to you."

"Will Daddy suffer?"

Behind the door, he shakes his head.

This is the end for a patient and friend.

COMPOSURE
SHAINA MAGNESS (CRS JULY 2021)

His last visit was over three years ago and today he enters in a hospital wheelchair, complaining of knee pain and swollen legs.

Back then, tests showed his kidneys were starting to fail, yet he stayed away.

Feet swollen to the size of cantaloupes, calves as thick as thighs, and toes necrotic.

Untreated kidney disease and diabetes.

Calmly, Dr. F says to the patient, "I would like to order some labs, then we can plan from there," then privately to me, "This will not end well."

THE PAST
ALEXIS HEAD (PRE-MATRIC JUNE 2023)

He didn't want anything to do with needles 6 months ago

"Should we try the injections now?"

"No" he responded

Okay.

"We can continue your current treatment."

He said, "That's fine but what medication for diabetes makes my friends lose weight?"

"It's the injections we talked about last visit"

"Great. Let's try those," He said.

TODAY
ALEXIS HEAD (PRE-MATRIC JUNE 2023)

She sat hunched over in a wheelchair.

Her daughter said, "Can you believe she carried her husband

down a ladder on her shoulder after an accident 10 years ago?"

Today, she has paper-thin skin.

Today, she is frail.

"She won't eat or drink."

Today, she is an 89-year-old woman.

She does not weigh 100 pounds.

ANNUAL VISIT
ALEXIS HEAD (PRE-MATRIC JUNE 2023)

He was the 4th patient that we had seen

for an annual visit.

His previous primary care physician had moved.

"I need my medications refilled," he said immediately after we walked in.

"Well, your labs look good. Do you have any concerns?"

"No," he said.

He only needed Cialis refilled.

The appointment lasted two minutes.

A LEADING HEART
ALEC TAYLOR (PRE-MATRIC JUNE 2023)

Covered in camo from head to toe, a rugged outdoorsman, he followed his heart and established an international career selling hunting gear. From China to Brazil, his heart led him across the globe. The downfall to his adventure will be his uncontrolled blood pressure and noncompliance. No more, will his heart be able to lead.

SMILING THROUGH THE PAIN
ALEC TAYLOR (PRE-MATRIC JUNE 2023)

Already 9 years old, but she had never attended school or interacted with kids before her grandmother gained custody. Her grandmother saved her from this horrific situation and comforts her through the frequent nightmares. I can only imagine her trauma. The provider recommended therapy, yet she still smiles through the pain.

SNOWBIRD
ALEC TAYLOR (PRE-MATRIC JUNE 2023)

Diagnosed with Cold agglutinin disease at 52, she is wary of leaving the house in the winter. Although she has this autoimmune disorder, she cracks jokes and maintains a good spirit. She says, "I have always wanted to become a snowbird anyways." We laughed and agreed that living on the beach beats hospitalizations.

DANCE AGAIN
ALEC TAYLOR (PRE-MATRIC JUNE 2023)

Diagnosed with lung cancer 2 weeks ago, the 70-year-old woman said she was a shell of her former self. She reminisced about her life and boasted about her youth, but she also regretted some eras of her life. Most of all, she wished her husband could take her dancing again.

LOSS OF IDENTITY
BRIAN HART (PRE-MATRIC JUNE 2023)

Is fifteen months enough to get over

losing someone so close? She was his caretaker

for the last nine years after the diagnosis, but his wife

for how many more than that before?

His fingerprint hangs around her neck, but she says

with him gone, it seems so is her identity. Who is she, really?

FAITH IN THE DARKNESS
BRIAN HART (PRE-MATRIC JUNE 2023)

The cancer has spread and multiple infections

attack her tired body. Her husband's congregation

is praying for healing. Even for those with a promise of

eternal life, the first death that comes to us all is too

daunting,

and the suggestion of a DNR elicits a

simple,

stoic,

"We're not going to think about that."

THE WEIGHT OF THE WORLD
BRIAN HART (PRE-MATRIC JUNE 2023)

She still manages to wear a smile, and

her laugh is infectious, even though

despite all she's trying,

her weight has gone up once again.

Behind the smile are feelings other than

happiness, so without consistent help from

someone to talk with to get the feelings out,

she takes them back in with a spoon.

TIME FOR CHANGE
BRIAN HART (PRE-MATRIC JUNE 2023)

You can see the pride on his face.

The doctor responds with a look of

pleasant surprise on hers and asks how

he did it.

He rolls up his sleeve to reveal the patch.

"After forty years, these ten days are the longest

I've gone without a cigarette."

He decided it was time for change.

ESTABLISHING CARE
COLLIN MCGLONE (PRE-MATRIC JUNE 2023)

"Alright, let's go."

She approached the patient room with me in tow.

I was excited, having only seen her work with patients that treat her as an
old friend.

A teenage girl sat on the table. She continued her FaceTime call during examination.

Anxiety, depression, ADHD. Multiple medications daily.

All while still being a child.

SANGUINITY
COLLIN MCGLONE (PRE-MATRIC JUNE 2023)

She lost her leg as a child.

She was overweight, a single mother, and had to move back in with her parents due to finances.

Who could blame her for being unhappy? Except she wasn't.

She warmly smiled while discussing her son, weight loss progress, and other family members.

Her contagious enthusiasm was extraordinarily inspiring.

HABITS
COLLIN MCGLONE (PRE-MATRIC JUNE 2023)

"Do you know where you are?" asked the nurse.

The man was slow to respond and slurred his answer.

This wasn't surprising, with 'alcoholic beverage' and lorazepam listed in his medications.

I prayed he would heal, but his advanced lung cancer made it unlikely.

Habits had caught up with him, and they weren't letting go.

PILL ORGANIZER
COLLIN MCGLONE (PRE-MATRIC JUNE 2023)

We talked about her blood pressure medication. Sometimes she forgets to take it.

That's understandable, maybe try a pill organizer?

Just like her husband had. His kidneys left him on a cocktail of drugs and dialysis before he passed.

I could only offer her a tissue and listen. That was all she needed from me.

her husband could take her dancing again.

THE PRETTIEST TEACHER IN SCHOOL
EMILY BOLINGER (PRE-MATRIC JUNE 2023)

"I remember her"

A third-grade boy behind a doctor's desk

and a student teacher in a cute skirt

"Howdy Mrs. Mae"

A third-grade boy in a doctor's coat

and a blushing student teacher

in a patient's seat

"Your sugar looks good"

A relieved patient smiles

at a distinguished physician

"You were the prettiest teacher in school"

Both smile in reminiscence.

PURPLE BLUE EYES
EMILY BOLINGER (PRE-MATRIC JUNE 2023)

Her voice sounded rough

Like hearing sandpaper

Head to toe in purple

Fixed up to see the do

"How are you today?"

Asks the doc

2 blue sparkling eyes directed at me,

the student,

As helpless

as the diamonds cutting through me

"If you can't help me

I'm gonna die"

At least she'd go out in style

PERFECT STORM
EMILY BOLINGER (PRE-MATRIC JUNE 2023)

I was told about the patient in room 2

One of *those* people

Who had gone through the storm

I entered the room

searching for his scars

But saw someone

sitting in a ball cap

with a laugh that was contagious

I realized

He was one of *those* people

Who survived the perfect storm

PATIENTS LIE??
EMILY BOLINGER (PRE-MATRIC JUNE 2023)

The nurse peeked into the office

"She booked for back pain

But her back is fine today"

It was never her back

"I had to put some reason"

Turns out

It was her heart

She couldn't see her internal mess

In one word on a screen

Why do patients lie?

Why can't doctors fly?

SEEKING CHANGE TODAY
HOPE DULL-POTTER (PRE-MATRIC JUNE 2023)

He spoke in a series of "yes" and "no sir". Meth, alcohol, and admission of guilt plagued the man who shuffled after every uncomfortable question. Married six times, but no children. A baby brother murdered by age thirty. He shook our hands as he left. He wore blue disposable scrubs and yellow hospital socks.

HAVE YOU HEARD THE NEWS?
HOPE DULL-POTTER (PRE-MATRIC JUNE 2023)

A right hip pain worked into a full schedule. The doctor smiled and said, "Does that sound like a good plan?" She started to cry. "Have you heard the news?" A sixteen-year-old grandson killed two weeks prior. A sister who passed away two months ago. Ah, that is why she presents today.

MY FRIEND'S MOM
HOPE DULL-POTTER (PRE-MATRIC JUNE 2023)

She was the doctor's high school teacher's wife. Her friend's mom. A member of the same local church. All the results came back good. By the end, both were in laughter reminiscing of childhood stories. As the doctor was leaving she said, "We need to catch up outside of the office."

SHARED SORROW
HANNAH TURNER (PRE-MATRIC JUNE 2023)

"How is your nephew?"

Eyes full of sorrow threaten to spill tears

Her nephew is in critical condition. ECMO was discontinued.

He is 6 weeks old.

Tears flow.

I am an auntie too.

I blink back tears.

The attending moves on with the visit.

My mind struggles to pay attention.

My eyes eventually clear.

TREMORS
HANNAH TURNER (PRE-MATRIC JUNE 2023)

Shaking hands. Shaking speech.

Shaking hope.

Her brain stem is wasting away, but we don't know why.

Neurologists shake their heads.

"Maybe the big city doctors can help you"

Her body is shaking, failing to support everyday activities.

Her mind is clear.

She knows we can't fix it.

She is tired of shaking.

SWIMMING
HANNAH TURNER (PRE-MATRIC JUNE 2023)

"I haven't been doing my shoulder exercises" confessed the patient, her eyes downcast.

"Have you done any other exercise?"

"I like getting in the pool at the Y" she said, her eyes igniting with enthusiasm.

Her blouse caught my attention with waves of blue and green, and I couldn't help but smile.

She left with a treatment plan of water aerobics instead of shoulder exercises.

TREASURES
HANNAH TURNER (PRE-MATRIC JUNE 2023)

A little boy sat on the exam table, his blue eyes focused on the trains by his side.

"Which one is Thomas?" I ask, crouching.

"This one" he whispers, holding up a treasured blue train.

His Grandma gently played with him as she told us that she was his guardian as he had been abandoned by both parents.

He was no longer abandoned.

He was treasured.

SMOKING
JORDAN HARBIN (PRE-MATRIC JUNE 2023)

Black lung. Emphysema. COPD. Asthma.

Established 90 seconds after walking in.

Rail thin, save for a big barrel chest.

"Could you just quit?" the doctor asked.

"Could you just shoot me?"

Vaping is bad, but not as bad as cigarettes.

"I heard vaping shreds your lungs."

On lunch I saw him leaving a gas station.

SLOW DAY
JORDAN HARBIN (PRE-MATRIC JUNE 2023)

We've seen 3 patients between 8:00 and 1:00.

4 other appointments were no shows.

A man came in with a bullet fragment lodged near his spine.

The complaint was back pain,

Then arm weakness,

Then his knees.

The affected side changed often during the interview.

It was almost interesting, and he skipped his last MRI

HIDING THE TRUTH
JORDAN HARBIN (PRE-MATRIC JUNE 2023)

Being a medical student feels like you're in the way.

His newly diagnosed diabetes was under control.

The depression he felt after his dad passed had gotten a lot better.

Taking the "pretend" patient history felt inane,

but it is necessary to develop the skill.

This guy was doing alright.

Then, the doctor came in.

DIFFERENT DEFINITIONS
JORDAN HARBIN (PRE-MATRIC JUNE 2023)

The patient is here for anxiety.

I know anxiety.

Panic, no rational thoughts, prove I'm not having a heart attack or an aneurysm.

I cannot die.

Naturally, I'm interested in her presentation.

"My eye has been twitching for like two weeks now.

I started teaching kindergarten and you know, I just need to mellow out…"

CHECK OUT
LAUREN TROUT (PRE-MATRIC JUNE 2023)

"This may be the first patient I have to write *thyroid cancer* on his death certificate."

One cancer treatment is causing other types of cancer. He's already had a tracheotomy and refuses another one. Even if it's the only thing to save his life.

"I guess I'll just check out then," through strained breaths.

CAN'T ARGUE WITH JESUS
LAUREN TROUT (PRE-MATRIC JUNE 2023)

She needed surgery that could result in a complete hysterectomy. She could've been referred to a specialist that may not have had to take it.

She wanted her own baby so bad, even though she knew the risks of a geriatric pregnancy.

"Jesus sent me to you, I want you to do it."

You can't argue with Jesus.

IT'S NOT FOR WEIGHT LOSS
LAUREN TROUT (PRE-MATRIC JUNE 2023)

He had strong opinions about nearly everything. They were especially strong regarding people using his diabetes medicine for weight loss.

"Why can't they just diet exercise? I need this to stay alive, they're just lazy."

Sometimes the people need a little help to kick start the weight loss then the diet and exercise helps.

COUNTRY REDNECK
LAUREN TROUT (PRE-MATRIC JUNE 2023)

He introduced himself to me by referring to himself as a "country redneck." He managed his type 1 diabetes well for just being a country redneck. He got good at estimating his insulin dosages with each meal, but the pump could do it so much better.

"I'm good with the needles, but I can if I have to."

FIRST DAY
LINDSAY TUCKER (PRE-MATRIC JUNE 2023)

It's my first time speaking to a patient alone and my heart is racing. As the sweet woman looked at me with teary eyes explaining the overwhelming stress that comes from caring for her sick mother, all of my nerves disappeared and humanity took over. I learned it isn't always medicine that our patients need.

CONCERNS
LINDSAY TUCKER (PRE-MATRIC JUNE 2023)

Dental work is not a typical reason to see a PCP, but that is what got her in after twenty years of not seeing a doctor. Hypertension that needs to be controlled before her dentist will proceed is the patient's biggest concern. However, the two golf ball sized masses brought up as an afterthought, quickly became the physicians.

CIRRHOSIS
LINDSAY TUCKER (PRE-MATRIC JUNE 2023)

Twenty-two liters of fluid were removed from the abdomen in the last three weeks for this newly established patient. As much as the doctor wanted to get to know the man sitting in front of her, there were more pressing matters at hand. The patient's tired eyes told us he was ready for answers not introductions.

A CHAMPION
THOMAS PATRICK (PRE-MATRIC JUNE 2023)

I mentioned medical school and was told "you're not gonna learn unless you see the sick ones." Sick was putting her condition mildly, but she never let it dull her spirit.

"My PT is done and I'm gonna continue to do it from home" she exclaimed. All I could think was "Man, what a champ."

AORTIC VALVE REPLACEMENT
THOMAS PATRICK (PRE-MATRIC JUNE 2023)

I look at the next patient, "Aortic Valve Replacement". My curiosity peaked.

Like a ping pong ball bouncing down a staircase, it sounded to me like the rhythm of her heart was off. "lub whoosh, dub" I could hear from the stethoscope. "Her murmur can be heard from the door" The doctor said light heartedly.

CHEESEBURGER
THOMAS PATRICK (PRE-MATRIC JUNE 2023)

"Your blood pressure is still high, are you taking those medications like I asked you?" The doctor asked.

She then exclaimed "I do the same thing every week, every day, every minute, and every second. I have got my medicine down."

"Well you must be eating an extra cheeseburger then." the doctor jokes with her.

3 WEEKS SOBER
THOMAS PATRICK (PRE-MATRIC JUNE 2023)

First thing I heard when we walked into the room was, "I relapsed, I did meth."

As the doctor talked with her about the substance abuse, the patient reassured she was turning things around. "Now I am sober! I have a job, I am clean and I have been going to church for 3 weeks."

A MOTHER'S LOVE
TALIA WOODRUFF (PRE-MATRIC JUNE 2023)

"I want a VBAC," expressed the mother. The doctor explained that VBAC was an option but does have pros and cons, especially after her two C-section children. "I just want to hold my baby first." After the fear was determined, the doctor reassured her that she would hold the baby first barring any complications.

QUITTING TOO LATE
TALIA WOODRUFF (PRE-MATRIC JUNE 2023)

The doctor strolled in with me slowly following. She lit up when we entered. She had her feet ready to be examined due to her diabetes when she exclaimed, "I want to quit smoking." We were ecstatic until the doctor examined her feet and she had no feeling at all.

ECHO
TALIA WOODRUFF (PRE-MATRIC JUNE 2023)

As we entered the room, the usually rambunctious patient lay on the exam table asleep. Her grandmother beside her. They had come to get a physical for a sleep study prescribed by the ENT specialist. Her breathing was audibly labored due to tonsils so enlarged. The sound echoed in the small room.

BLAME THE ARMY
TALIA WOODRUFF (PRE-MATRIC JUNE 2023)

The jolly man sat on the exam table wondering who I was. After introducing myself I started into my list of questions. His arthritis was bothering him from head to knee. As I looked fascinatingly on, he explained that the Army was the culprit. Thank you, CB, for your service.

URGENT CARE
ALEXIS HEAD (PRE-MATRIC JUNE 2023)

"Hey doc my arm is messed up"

His wrist was the size of a baseball.

He couldn't bend it.

"I think I have gout"

"Why do you think that? Have you ever had bloodwork?"

"No" the patient responded.

"Do you have a primary care doctor?"

"Yes, but I have never made an appointment with her."

HEMORRHOIDS
ALEXIS HEAD (PRE-MATRIC JUNE 2023)

He was in pain sitting down.

"I've been sitting on this donut because it hurts to sit down."

"I've had hemorrhoids before, and I think I just need more suppositories."

The nurse practitioner looked and said, "oh yes that's hemorrhoids."

"Hopefully I'll be able to sit down at the MLB game I'm going to tomorrow."

VOICEMAIL
ALEXIS HEAD (PRE-MATRIC JUNE 2023)

The doctor had just received her lab results.

Her bloodwork shows that she has Hepatitis C.

He dialed her phone number.

Voicemail.

The doctor left a message.

"Please call me back, this is a treatable disease in 2023."

He was clearly distraught after leaving multiple voicemails delivering the news.

She has yet to call back

COLONOSCOPY
ALEXIS HEAD (PRE-MATRIC JUNE 2023)

"I did that Cologuard"

The doctor responded, "I see that and think we need to set up a colonoscopy."

The patient finally said,

"FedEx didn't ship it within the instruction time. That's why the results were positive"

The doctor explained the significance of his results.

"I don't want a colonoscopy," the patient responded.

HYPERTENSION
ALEXIS HEAD (PRE-MATRIC JUNE 2023)

The patient's blood pressure had been high.

The nurse practitioner asked, "what's going on?"

"My daughter got in a car accident."

"One brother is in the psychiatric hospital."

"The other brother is drinking again."

"But work is stress free."

The patient explained that he works at the local prison in the substance abuse department.

PALLIATIVE CARE
ALEXIS HEAD (PRE-MATRIC JUNE 2023)

"I have sepsis."

This patient has been to the ER five times in the past 2 months.

The APRN called back, "What's going on?"

He listed off concerns the next 15 minutes.

"Thanks for listening, I'll go to the ER if I have a fever," the patient said.

He hung up without the APRN's response

PARTY ANIMAL
ALEC TAYLOR (PRE-MATRIC JUNE 2023)

Her friends considered her a party animal in her youth. Now 36, she says her alcohol use has ruined her life. It began with her DUI, but now she picks between sobriety and sleeping. She cries, "Doc, can you give me something to help me sleep? I don't want to drink anymore." Proper sleep heals.

AFRAID TO TELL SOMEONE
ALEC TAYLOR (PRE-MATRIC JUNE 2023)

Restricted to a wheelchair and a victim of several comorbidities, the middle-aged woman had horrid physical health. Now a victim of sexual assault, her mental health has deteriorated. Afraid to tell anyone else about the incident but she trusts her provider. Teary-eyed, she confides this traumatic experience to her nurse practitioner. Empathetic connections matter.

I KNOW BETTER
ALEC TAYLOR (PRE-MATRIC JUNE 2023)

As a former nurse, he used to witness the effects of patients not complying with their medications. Now with an A1C of 9.5, he says, "I know better, but I have stressors in my life that contribute to my noncompliance." You can lead a horse to water but cannot make it drink.

GARDEN GIFTS
ALEC TAYLOR (PRE-MATRIC JUNE 2023)

He complained he had to leave his garden to come in. Nevertheless, he smiled and greeted his doctor with a firm handshake. The medications have controlled his hypertension and diabetes. He lost weight too. At the end of the visit, he gifts his doctor fresh garden cucumbers and tomatoes. This epitomizes an optimal physician-patient relationship.

SEEING CRITTERS
ALEC TAYLOR (PRE-MATRIC JUNE 2023)

Diagnosed with insomnia after not sleeping a wink in years, she has tried several medications. She has tired eyes. She says, "This new medicine has me seeing critters." Her options for treatment are limited. She cries, "I want to sleep again." The doctor pats her on the back. She is referred to a sleep clinic.

OVERLOADED
BRIAN HART (PRE-MATRIC JUNE 2023)

The newest patient to the office sat there in

the wheelchair, her head bowed

down with the weight of the years.

with every new issue her caretaker

brought up, she'd chide, "Now, we don't

want to overload him with that on the first day."

She couldn't acknowledge that it was she,

who was overloaded

THE LOST HALF
BRIAN HART (PRE-MATRIC JUNE 2023)

She sits stoically, her upper lip stiff

and her cheeks dry, but her lower lip betrays a quiver,

and her eyes glisten with held back tears.

His heart has only been silent for a month.

She has regained her shed weight

and increased the number of cigarettes,

to try making up for her lost half.

CROSSING THAT LINE
BRIAN HART (PRE-MATRIC JUNE 2023)

He speaks with so much passion

about leaving his reality,

going back to college,

and playing collegiate sports:

"Just gotta start makin' good decisions to

get across that line."

But how do you tell someone with 44 years,

in that kind of health, his fantasy is just that,

without crossing the line?

COMMITMENT
COLLIN MCGLONE (PRE-MATRIC JUNE 2023)

Her memory had recently begun declining. As her husband asked me about school, she gave me a friendly smile from the exam table.

He brought all her medications and his cane.

His cancer had come back, but he was confident he'd win.

I believed him.

For 55 years, they had taken care of each other.

CLINGING ON
COLLIN MCGLONE (PRE-MATRIC JUNE 2023)

I hoped my face did not reveal my shock when seeing the man. His skeletal figure barely filled the wheelchair.

His lungs in shambles, he depended on oxygen. He also still depended on cigarettes; he pointed out the burn on his face.

He knew they will kill him, but they were all he still enjoyed.

CAN'T SLOW DOWN
COLLIN MCGLONE (PRE-MATRIC JUNE 2023)

"So, doc, can I get back to dancing?" asked the smiling, slender man with a full head of hair.

He got his approval and recommended we both come watch him soon.

"I can really burn up that dance floor" he remarked with a flurry of foot taps, casting doubt on his listed age of 86.

GLASS HALF FULL
COLLIN MCGLONE (PRE-MATRIC JUNE 2023)

On paper, she was bound to crutches, permanently used a Foley catheter, and had gotten a *C. diff.* infection again.

With her smiling, joke cracking, and palpable energy, you would think nothing was wrong.

Her cards would have made many a cynic, but she was one of the folks who didn't seem to get down.

WISE
EMILY BOLINGER (PRE-MATRIC JUNE 2023)

She was sweet

And young

Excited to show her vacation pictures

And her new cat

"She is helping me take my mind off of it"

Her house had just burnt down

"Do you think about hurting yourself?"

"I promised my mom I would never do that

I couldn't leave her like this"

I looked into her eyes,

wise beyond her years

I WANNA, I NEEDA
EMILY BOLINGER (PRE-MATRIC JUNE 2023)

"I'm in misery at all times"

She has been raising her adult kid's kids

"I'm on the edge"

Why doesn't she step back?

"I wanna wring everyone's neck"

"I'm gonna jump off the cliff"

Because her daughter has threatened to take the kids away

"I wanna wring my neck"

"I needa Valium"

"Please"

NO TEETH, ALL LAUGHS
EMILY BOLINGER (PRE-MATRIC JUNE 2023)

When you hear it,

You can't help but smile

When you hear it

You see her missing teeth

4 whole teeth missing in the front

When you hear it,

You forget her history of drug abuse

When you hear it,

She becomes a human being

When you hear it,

You want her to get better.

SIMPLE ENOUGH-EMILY BOLINGER (PRE-MATRIC JUNE 2023)

Face down on the weighted bed

I knew she didn't wanna talk

Especially about her episode

So I asked about her favorite music instead

"Life is a Highway is my favorite"

She cracked a smile

I did too and asked

"What would make life better?"

"I want to be near my family"

That's all.

THE DONUT
EMILY BOLINGER (PRE-MATRIC JUNE 2023)

I have never seen one before

In picture nor in person

I waited in the corner

Eyes diverting around the room

Leaning over a shoulder

The duck bill showed me where to look

It sat there in plain sight

As if for me to place my order

"I'll have the round and pink one"

I HAVE THE SNEEZES
HOPE DULL-POTTER (PRE-MATRIC JUNE 2023)

Dogs, cats, and a variety of trees. The doctor showed him his allergy sensitivity results. "I don't know how you keep all those animals and trees with how allergic you are to them." He sneezed. "I think I'm allergic to 'V'." The doctor turned to me and said, "'V' is his wife."

DON'T JUDGE A BOOK BY ITS COVER
HOPE DULL-POTTER (PRE-MATRIC JUNE 2023)

He was 6'4. He wore Harley Davidson earrings. He had long hair pulled back in a low ponytail. His A1C was below 7. He not only logged every sugar, but every insulin injection. The doctor told him he was a responsible patient. The man rode all the way to hear the doctor's praises and encouragement.

IT DOESN'T MATTER WHAT IT COSTS
HOPE DULL-POTTER (PRE-MATRIC JUNE 2023)

It was her diabetic shoes that brought her into the office. It was the pain in her back that caused the tears. She yelled for her husband's help after struggling for thirty minutes to get out of the bathtub on her own. He mouths the words, "It doesn't matter what it costs."

CONFIDENTIAL STUFF
HOPE DULL-POTTER (PRE-MATRIC JUNE 2023)

Her eyes were wet as we walked in the room. She said, "I'm sorry. This is the first time I've had a minute to myself." Her husband. Leukemia. An estranged son. She said, "I'm sorry to ramble on." The doctor said, "Please talk to me. Who else would you talk to?" She said, "No one."

I'M LEAVING, I'VE GOT THINGS TO DO
HOPE DULL-POTTER (PRE-MATRIC JUNE 2023)

Non-compliant. The doctor knew what the next room held before we walked in. He was 80 years old, head bent over on his walker. He said, "I feel like crap." A smoker. A diabetic. The doctor showed him the medicines he didn't pick up at the pharmacy. The patient left before the visit was over.

ARE YOU PROUD OF YOURSELF?
HOPE DULL-POTTER (PRE-MATRIC JUNE 2023)

The doctor and I walked in. It was a woman and daughter sitting in the room. The doctor calculated the results on a calculator on her phone. She held it up to the patient. "You are down 13 pounds since the medicine. Are you proud of yourself?" The patient cried and shook her head "yes".

SCREENING
HANNAH TURNER (PRE-MATRIC JUNE 2023)

The patient's twinkling eyes, quick laughter, and full beard reminded me of St. Nick. His swollen and encrusted ankles confirmed his reported diabetes.

We happily conversed as I put little drops of his blood on a testing strip.

Another student worked on connecting him with a doctor.

He walked away with a smile, knowing he would soon have a doctor again.

"RETIREMENT"
HANNAH TURNER (PRE-MATRIC JUNE 2023)

"I can only sit around the house and yard so long!" Observed the newly retired truck driver.

He was here to get his the physical for trucking license renewal.

Excitement to start work part-time again radiated from him.

I couldn't help but celebrate with him.

LOSS
HANNAH TURNER (PRE-MATRIC JUNE 2023)

The frail old lady had suddenly lost her son. She was devastated.

"I've lost three children now, one when she was only seven. Drunk driver at Kroger. Only got one child left" she lamented through tears.

How had she had weathered so many losses? How could we even respond?

Listening, Empathy, Medication.

Prayer.

The lady's eyes calmed a little after her nurse practitioner's prayer.

THE CHAIN
HANNAH TURNER (PRE-MATRIC JUNE 2023)

The middle-aged farmer wasn't breathing well. His airways felt clogged.

His mother had offered him opiates to help him breath. He got hooked.

Allergies to asthma to opiate addiction.

The chain could have been stopped so easily.

It took my breath away.

SMILES
HANNAH TURNER (PRE-MATRIC JUNE 2023)

"I've never felt happy like this! I have been depressed since I was 11!" Exclaimed the elderly lady, her whole face smiling.

After years of depression, an effective treatment had been found.

Excitement permeated the exam room.

After leaving the room, the NP's smile didn't fade.

"These cases make it worth it" she beamed.

NOW WHAT?
JORDAN HARBIN (PRE-MATRIC JUNE 2023)

"In the evening my tongue blisters and it burns from my esophagus to my vagina."

Hmm.

She's seen about every specialist in existence,

Has regular appointments with two or three other doctors.

No one's found it yet.

Physical exam is unremarkable.

She wants help, but also wants to stop taking all of her medicines.

Hmm.

NOT THIS TIME
JORDAN HARBIN (PRE-MATRIC JUNE 2023)

A scope is recommended every 5 years.

He already had kidney cancer.

"My father had colon cancer. My brother had leukemia. Sister died of breast cancer."

He seemed preoccupied; he wasn't present.

Some people go to the ED with a cold, then there's him.

He needed his Tylenol 4 refilled, and his depression was better.

"HUH?"
JORDAN HARBIN (PRE-MATRIC JUNE 2023)

"If I can't hear you just draw me a picture" she yelled.

"I'm 86 years old!"

The doctor explained that testing had indicated her hearing issues wouldn't be helped with hearing aids.

"I'm not wasting my money on hearing aids!"

She snatched the test results to read over them herself.

"My hearing is just fine!"

WAITING
JORDAN HARBIN (PRE-MATRIC JUNE 2023)

We were there with palliative care, the consult came over the weekend.

The room was surprisingly cheery considering the circumstances.

The wife had recently elected for hospice care in their home.

The wife and daughter sat there waiting, waiting to go home so they could wait for the end.

He didn't even look that sick.

THANK YOU, DOCTOR
JORDAN HARBIN (PRE-MATRIC JUNE 2023)

"I explain to my patients all the time that I'm not a doctor."

Said the APRN.

"Unless you earn your doctorate, then they **better** call you doctor!"

Said the NP student.

"I'm glad I don't think like that."

Said the APRN.

I'm very uncomfortable, I wish the next patient was here.

Thought the medical student.

DID HE KNOW?
LAUREN TROUT (PRE-MATRIC JUNE 2023)

Going through his box of medications, the nurse uncovered an unsettling pest. I don't know if it was good or bad judgment that she didn't tell us right away; she waited until he was out of ear shot.

She informed us of the numerous bed bugs found. Four rooms in the small clinic were shut down.

Meanwhile I'm wondering, "Did he know?"

THE ROBOT
LAUREN TROUT (PRE-MATRIC JUNE 2023)

The young doctor was the only one in ENT that knew how to use the new, fancy robot for complicated surgeries. So she examined the new patient with cancer growing in the back of his throat.

"We used to have to break the jaw bones to get to places like this. With the robot, recovery time is so much better."

THINNING OUT
LAUREN TROUT (PRE-MATRIC JUNE 2023)

Walking in, it was immediately obvious he had been crying. After examining his previous weights, he's significantly thinner than the last visit. His wife's passing really took a toll on him after being married for 60+ years. He was thinning out in more ways than one.

For no particular reason, the doctor requested a visit every 4 weeks.

NURSING HOME
LAUREN TROUT (PRE-MATRIC JUNE 2023)

He has fallen and fell asleep with a cigarette in his hand and burnt his leg severely. His wife had been doing the wound care, but it wasn't getting any better. It appeared infected when the physician looked at it.

After several fractures and superficial injuries, his wife was ready to put him in a nursing home. She couldn't keep "babysitting" him.

DONE
LAUREN TROUT (PRE-MATRIC JUNE 2023)

For the new inpatient evaluation, he was already asked so many questions. His wife answered most things for him because he did not want to cooperate at all.

By the time it was my turn to interview him, he was absolutely over the questions. He did not say a word. "I'm ready to get the hell out of here," was the only answer I got.

GETTING BACK UP
LINDSAY TUCKER (PRE-MATRIC JUNE 2023)

Since turning thirty, a dark cloud has hovered over her. An urgent spinal surgery, Crohn's disease diagnosis, and severe motorcycle accident is enough to keep anyone down. "I knew if I didn't get back up and try, I would suffer in my own pity." Today, you would never be able to tell how much she had overcome.

SECOND CHANCE
LINDSAY TUCKER (PRE-MATRIC JUNE 2023)

His pain management started with prescribed pills, then they weren't, then he added alcohol. His life was falling apart. At his lowest moment, he grabbed his gun and pulled the trigger. Nothing happened, he was alive, and his only explanation was the Lord. That lowest day was actually the first of his second chance.

A DATE AT THE DOCTOR
LINDSAY TUCKER (PRE-MATRIC JUNE 2023)

The visit was full of snarky comments, soft smiles, and head shakes. This couple had been married for over forty years. They answered the doctor's questions for each other much more than they did for themselves. I left the room grinning, hoping one day I was lucky enough to have a date at the doctor.

WORLD
LINDSAY TUCKER (PRE-MATRIC JUNE 2023)

"Spell world backwards." "D L R O W" is what we expected but instead we got a confused glance, stuttering, and eventually an "I don't know." Could it be that she had early onset dementia like her mother? Or maybe it was a lack of education. Or rather, the fact that two medical students she had never met are grilling her with questions. How do you decipher?

THE YOUNG ONES
LINDSAY TUCKER (PRE-MATRIC JUNE 2023)

Innocent blue eyes and a toothy smile looked up at me as I entered the room. You would never be able to guess this little boy had been through harder trials in his two years of life than I've ever been close to in my twenty-two. His mother in jail for child abuse and his father nowhere to be seen, I think of how hard it will be to care for children like him knowing I can't change the cards they've been dealt.

REMOVING SUTURES
THOMAS PATRICK (PRE-MATRIC JUNE 2023)

As I put on my gloves, the physician showed me how to properly remove sutures. Using her guidance, I began removing the sutures one by one.

I was so happy to get to do something hands on. In the end, the patient was really happy with the results, which is all I could ask for.

MUHLENBERG COUNTY
THOMAS PATRICK (PRE-MATRIC JUNE 2023)

As I traveled on the Western Kentucky Parkway, I remember my father telling me there was a song about Muhlenberg County. I looked out at the land. I realized I didn't have much longer in this beautiful place and just like the person singing the song, I would be yearning to come back here soon.

BE LIKE HER
THOMAS PATRICK (PRE-MATRIC JUNE 2023)

Every time I ask patients what they believe makes a great doctor, they always reply with "just be like Dr W."

I was ending my session with an older lady when she answered with "make your patients feel like you care. Dr W does this so well that I think of her like my own sister.

THE IDEAL PATIENT
THOMAS PATRICK (PRE-MATRIC JUNE 2023)

"Check and check your test results are great. How much weight have you lost?" the doctor says.

"I was 270 and now I'm 155. Also, I am down to 5 cigarettes a day." the patient exclaims.

"What's your secret" I ask

"Stop snacking, eat healthy-ish and walk often." she replies.

All while tapering cigarettes? Bravo.

SIMPLE MAN
THOMAS PATRICK (PRE-MATRIC JUNE 2023)

He talked about his time with the military in Vietnam. He loved the outdoors and tending to cattle. He was a simple man, one of the last few true cowboys.

He said "always remember, you can learn something from everyone. I don't like me, myself and I people. I like we, our and us people."

LIVING TO SEE HIS FIRST CHILD –TALIA
WOODRUFF (PRE-MATRIC JUNE 2023)

The man looked old and worn. He turned out to be 33 years old and was diagnosed with metastatic colon cancer a year ago. His wife was due in August with their first child, and they talked like lovers about wanting more. His healthcare team didn't believe he would live to see August.

A BLUR
TALIA WOODRUFF (PRE-MATRIC JUNE 2023)

The doctor explained that tinnitus is common prior to walking in the room but as the man was examined there was a blur between if the inner ear was causing it or his Atrial fibrillation. With 2 swift moves akin to a baptism it was determined to be his Atrial fibrillation.

USELESS HANDS
TALIA WOODRUFF (PRE-MATRIC JUNE 2023)

I heard her coming before I saw her. The patients' loud raspy voice squealed as she held her hands out in front of her. She cried "I can't do nothing with these hands." The arthritis in her hands had caused the fingers to be stuck and painful with movement.

DRINKING
TALIA WOODRUFF (PRE-MATRIC JUNE 2023)

The man shook my hand as I was introduced as the student observing. He seemed vibrant and happy and even showed me a picture of his cabin at Pennyrile. Afterwards the doctor mentioned that he might've been drinking to account for the shakiness and dementia was not far.

NOT DOING WELL
TALIA WOODRUFF (PRE-MATRIC JUNE 2023)

The patient sat on the table with long brown hair and a bright blue dress. She started in on how she was taking an antidepressant, but it decreased her libido, and her husband noticed it. The patient started crying and explained that she wasn't doing well after coming off the Effexor.

HEARING AIDS
JACK DODDS (CRS JULY 2023)

He was losing his hearing in his old age.

He had the most expensive hearing aids,

His family bought them for him.

They were not helping.

We had to yell for him to hear us.

The doctor told him that they only worked if he wore them

"Yeah I should probably take them out of the box"

TRAVEL
JACK DODDS (CRS JULY 2023)

One hour and fifteen minutes,

Two hours and thirty minutes,

Forty-five minutes, and one hour.

Of the eight patients we saw,

Four had traveled over an hour.

They had no choice,

Without care for their diabetes, they would die.

Without making that drive, they would suffer.

But they couldn't get that care closer to home.

LIFE TO THE FULLEST
KATE KELLER (CRS JULY 2023)

The doctor warned me of this patient before we saw him, He called him "Grumpy," He seemed more worried to me, though, How am I doing with my blood sugar, doc? He asked. Maybe he wasn't worried, just curious. "A friend told me I should stop jet skiing, but you don't think I should, do you?" The doc shook his head and laughed, "No" he said, "Keep on living life to the fullest." "That's what I plan on doing," he said.

NOT THE SAME
KATE KELLER (CRS JULY 2023)

A pair of sunglasses rested on his eyes, The left side of his face drooped, A 'halfway' smile was all he could give, A sudden shock this was to him, That his life might be changed forever, Yet he said, "I really don't like drinking my beer out of a straw, it's just not the same." He had no control over the left side of his face, And his main concern was that he couldn't drink his beer the same way.

CLASS CLOWN
AUBREY KNOP (CRS JULY 2023)

As soon as you walked into the room his personality shined.

A huge smile spread across his face that was accompanied by jokes that cracked up the whole room. However, the words started to slur.

Stroke?

No, thankfully.

Bell's Palsy.

His mouth drooped, forehead resembled one that had Botox in it, and his eye remained open.

But the jokes never stopped.

STRANGER
AUBREY KNOP (CRS JULY 2023)

A raspy voice boomed through the hallway and found a way to our ears.

Soon, a tiny body approached that occupied that powerful voice.

The stranger.

He came in with a wide smile and bright eyes. He struggled to speak but that did not kinder his spirit.

His joy made everyone in the office smile.

Every hospital needs a stranger.

ON BOTH ENDS
ISAAC KREBS (CRS JULY 2023)

Today I started, faced with the end. Not the giving up part, but the hard part indeed. She knew something I did not, peace. I silently observed. Small talk is large, body language is everything. We now know how to help, to do for her what she can't. I can't wait for the wonders ahead.

NOT OUR FIRST RODEO
IAN LEATHERMAN (CRS JULY 2023)

Patient has been diagnosed with stage 3 stomach cancer. Today is her first day of chemotherapy. Her hands are clasped tightly in between her thighs. "I am just nervous about this bein' my first time" He places his hand on her back. "It is your first time, but it most definitely is not ours.

ANTARCTICA
JESSICA LEWIS (CRS JULY 2023)

She was wheeled into the OR and started shaking

uncontrollably from the suffocation of cold air.

As the betadine was applied to her stomach,

she went from shaking due to the cold to shaking from her laughter.

When words could not calm her down,

the tickling sensation of the betadine on her stomach did.

The climate in the room changed from Antarctica to California.

BEST WE CAN DO
MADISON PAYNE (CRS JULY 2023)

When a patient is sick, we try to provide the best treatment.

When it is as simple as taking your medicine every day and coming in for checkups.

The "I forgot" or "I didn't want to take that one medication."

We just want them to feel better.

There is only so much we can do.

WEAKENING HEART
MADISON PAYNE (JULY 2023)

60 days from diagnosis to death.

All that's left is a weakening heart and four girls without a mother.

Is the appetite gone or is it the food she would cook?

Has it been 7 months?

As the light of 52 years of marriage vanishes from his eyes, he still uses the word "we".

MIRROR
SYDNEY SHOULDERS (CRS JULY 2023)

I was impressed by the twelve-year-old patient who sat before me.

She moved her ankle around like it hadn't been broken at all. Never even winced, not one facial expression. She was just excited to get back to softball.

It was like there was a mirror in front of me,

I saw my younger self.

BODY DYSMORPHIA
COLE WELLS (CRS JULY 2023)

When your reflection turns traitor,

It's hard not to believe its deception.

If only you could see the person I see when I look at you.

I can't promise this will be an easy journey,

But I'm confident that one day you will look in the mirror and smile at the person looking back at you.

THE SOLDIER
ISAAC KREBS (CRS JULY 2023)

It was a fight. No blood, no weapons. Much pain. With fists balled at my side, I watched the general strategize and sympathize with one of his brave soldiers sidelined by, for days on end, invisible misery. With rash symptoms showing and initial action taken, the enemy fought back hard. The soldier fought back harder.

SEE YOU AROUND
IAN LEATHERMAN (CRS JULY 2023)

The visit was wrapping up, the boy's foot was healed.

He was ready to start playing ball again.

"I don't want to see you guys around here any time soon," said the NP

"Hopefully not. We will see you at Kroger before we see you here again," said the father.

THE TRUST IN A PRIMARY CARE PROVIDER
SYDNEY SHOULDERS (CRS JULY 2023)

The nurse practitioner made each of her patient visits admiringly personable. We saw many patients, but the last was special.

The patient openly admitted to prescription drug abuse. She said, "I'm going to be completely honest with you because you're doing everything to get me right."

The trust in her primary care provider was powerful.

SPIDERMAN
JACK DODDS (CRS JULY 2023)

His mom scheduled an appointment because he had been bitten.

He was covered in hives,

Yet when he arrived he was in very high spirits.

He was wearing a Spiderman hat, shirt, and shoes.

"He was bitten by some insect"

"Not an insect, they have six legs, A SPIDER,

How else can I turn into Spiderman?"

COMPASSION
KATE KELLER (CRS JULY 2023)

The door opened,

The smell of smoke immediately filled the room,

A middle-aged man sat in the chair across from the doc,

The doc explained his need for a medical procedure,

A tear ran down his face,

The doc rested his hand on the patient's shoulder,

The gap was closed between provider and patient,

It was now just one human to another,

Compassion.

TRUE LOVE
AUBREY KNOP (CRS JULY 2023)

True love

He made me believe in it

His eyes sparkled every time he looked at her

He only spoke with admiration when discussing their life together

But then the tears started to stroll

He didn't realize that he would only have a few weeks left with his wife

Time is slipping away, but his love for her isn't.

I WON'T GIVE UP
KATELYN MATTINGLY CRS JULY 2023)

He was used to asking the questions. He was used to treating the patients.

He has so much more work to do, so much more life to live.

But treatments were failing. The cancer was metastasizing. They hit road-block after roadblock.

The doctor says if this doesn't work it is time to consider hospice.

Husband and wife now fighting for every hope of it all not ending too soon.

ESCAPE
COLE WELLS (CRS JULY 2023)

Suicidal idealizations

Anger building up

Filling up frustration and

Desperate for the suffering to end

"It feels like no one understands me doc"

The patient stormed out of the room after realizing nothing we could prescribe him would take away the pain. But together they found hope to carry on, one step at a time.

FEAR AND COMPASSION
NIKKI HARNAGE (CRS JULY 2023)

For once I wasn't the one obviously out of place in the exam room.

I felt like a hybrid between patient and doctor — a translator between funny accents and funny sayings.

I stayed quiet though, I wasn't needed after a minute or two.

Tears and a hand to the shoulder.

Fear and compassion are universally understood.

ENDLESS WOUND
NIKKI HARNAGE (CRS JULY 2023)

Was her spine in there? I couldn't see.

The hole in her neck seemed endless, an abyss of wispy gray hair.

Freshly washed! Her hair— not her wound.

We didn't know how it got there, neither did she.

Did it hurt? A pressure.

I didn't know how her head stayed on her shoulders, but it seemed stuck there.

PRECEPTING INTRODUCTION
IAN LEATHERMAN (CRS JULY 2023)

We walked into the room of the first patient.

"This is Ian Leatherman, he was the Indiana state champion for heading and heeling in 2022"

The husband and wife's gaze turned to me.

I smiled and nodded, "Nice to meet you"

They turned back to Dr. F

"He actually hasn't ridden a horse a day in his life"

We laugh and the visit rolls on.

RETURNING THE FAVOR
IAN LEATHERMAN (CRS JULY 2023)

The patient had a wound that hadn't healed for 3 years.

It had developed into skin cancer and needed to be removed.

"I just need this fixed doc."

"We will get it figured out, don't worry."

"You are my eighth doctor now."

"Does that mean I get a Christmas card?"

WHAT IS PRIVACY?
MADISON PAYNE (CRS JULY 2023)

A crowd for learning a routine, open for all to view.

Modesty only under a small sheet and stockings up to her knees.

Dismisses the room for a moment, for a question that wanted to be unheard.

What is privacy when you have already seen it all?

BARBIE STICKER
MADISON PAYNE (CRS JULY 2023)

As she fidgets in the seat, she holds her gaze up at me.

Mom concerned with family history.

The otoscope glowing in her ears as she picks at her Band-Aid.

It's only fluid, a sigh of relief, and follow up in 3 months.

A proper visit for a 4-year-old is finished with a Barbie sticker.

THE FRIENDLY DOC
SYDNEY SHOULDERS (CRS JULY 2023)

The cardiologist walked into each room and greeted every patient like they were best friends.

"Hey brother! How are you today?"

He sat within two feet of each patient and patted them on the back and gave fist bumps, even when they were new patients.

He was one of the friendliest doctors I had met.

DR. GRAVES
COLE WELLS (CRS JULY 2023)

The patient's heart sank when she heard her diagnosis.

"Grave's Disease"

Sensing her fear, the doctor put a reassuring hand on her shoulder. He explained that this disease is completely manageable with the right medication. It's simply named after the doctor that discovered it.

"You should have started with that," she said with a grin.

LIVING WILL
JACK DODDS (CRS JULY 2023)

"Do you know where you are sir?"

"I'm in the hospital"

"Do you know what city we are in?"

"Madisonville"

"Do you know what year it is?"

"2023"

"Do you know why you're in the hospital?"

"2023"

"No, sir, what illness brought you to the hospital"

"Uh, 2023"

We all smiled at him as we left the room, knowing he wasn't competent to sign his living will.

SMILE AND NOD
JACK DODDS (CRS JULY 2023)

"Now before we talk about my CPAP let me warn you about some things"

"Oh boy" went through my head

"Now I know doctors have god complexes and all, but don't drink the Kool-Aid"

"Vaccines are simply not good for you and I know because my father-in-law is a well-respected psychiatrist"

"Oh boy" went through my head

"And there is absolutely no reason for the Covid vaccine. I can treat Covid with my herbs from my living room"

"Oh boy" went through my head as I smiled and nodded my head.

3...2...1
JESSICA LEWIS
(CRS JULY 2023)

A family of

three waits in the exam room.

Two patients and

one mother.

When the doctor asks about a reason for the visit,

the mother quickly answers.

This is the pattern for the entirety of the visit.

The son is shy, but the daughter is independent.

She is like her mother in that way.

CIGARETTES
JESSICA LEWIS (CRS JULY 2023)

The smell of cigarette smoke is her natural scent.

Past heart issues and aneurysms

follow her around like the grim reaper.

She was hospitalized a month beforehand.

She pulls out a bag containing

six new medications she was prescribed.

Her ankles are the size of her legs.

She will probably smoke on her way home.

ONE THING LEADS TO ANOTHER
KATELYN MATTINGLY (CRS JULY 2023)

He came in for what he thought would be a quick trip to the hospital, an overnight stay at most. It has now been three weeks, three different rooms, and countless number of physicians.

"Do you know why you're in the hospital?" The nurse asked.

"2023" He responded.

What began with shortness of breath and fatigue has grown to a diagnosis of bladder cancer, anemia, confusion and more.

TRIAL AND ERROR
COLE WELLS (CRS JULY 2023)

"I don't want to take anything that doesn't make me feel like myself," said the patient

He asks the doctor if there was anything he could prescribe that would take away the pain. The last medication made things worse and the one before made him too tired.

The doctor reassured the patient that they would figure this out together. The patient trusted his doctor and hoped to find peace again soon.

LOVE REMAINED
KATE KELLER (CRS JULY 2023)

The lights flipped off,

On,

Off,

On,

Controlled by a five-year-old girl with autism,

Her language was actions, Her mother was tired,

Stressed,

Battered,

Bruised,

She needed answers,

The bite marks on her arm were marks from her daughter,

She loved her daughter, no doubt,

But her daughter was unable to express her love back to her,

A complicated relationship,

Controlled by lack of communication,

And yet,

After all the hurt,

Love remained

DIRT BIKES
KATE KELLER (CRS JULY 2023)

A love for dirt bikes,

Landed him a life flight,

His arms,

Now healed,

Once broken in two,

His leg,

Now strong,

Once fractured,

Now made new,

He detailed his fear,

Yet he had pulled through,

And 6 months later,

All he knew,

Was His love for dirt bikes,

He never outgrew.

EXPERIENCE IS CHANGE
ISAAC KREBS (CRS JULY 2023)

I woke up me, and I fell asleep Me. me listened to this boy, nearly my age, bare his soul about the horrors that changed him, and Me got up from that table changed by the real story of pain sitting 4 feet from me. That experience was a change for life, change for good.

CANCER "FREE"
SHAINA MAGNESS (PRE-CLINICAL JULY 2023)

"There is no clinical evidence that treatment longer than 5 years decreases further reoccurrence," the doctor explained. The patient's five years had finally come, she was breast cancer free, but she was scared to stop taking the pills. "Could you just feel this here, I've never noticed it before but isn't this a bump?" she asked.

SHE NEEDS TO SEE THIS
SHAINA MAGNESS (PRE-CLINICAL JULY 2023)

As the patient removed his pants he glanced nervously at me, "She's going to be a doctor, she needs to see this," the doctor reassured him. A fist-sized inguinal hernia, indirect, the doctor explained, meaning the patient's internal organs had traveled through a pre-formed canal towards his testicle, and reducible, the doctor continued as he pushed it back inside where it belonged.

DOWN
SHAINA MAGNESS (PRE-CLINICAL JULY 2023)

She said had been feeling real "down" lately, lower than she has been since before her "spa week" at the psychiatric unit last year. Her major depressive disorder drags her down, fed by life's daily stressors, until she can't find the energy to care for anything, even herself. Hopefully, a new prescription can help.

HER HEART
SHAINA MAGNESS (PRE-CLINICAL JULY 2023)

She was a busy woman, always on the go and taking care of others. Tests showed that her heart was beating too fast, averaging 105 beats per minute. Just like the woman herself, her left ventricle had trouble relaxing. Tearing up and fearing the worst, she asked what her condition meant in terms of life expectancy.

ADHD
RILEY ERIKSEN (PRE-CLINICAL JULY 2023)

In the exam room, a 12-year-old patient sat on the table with her mom in the chair beside her. When the mom brought up ADHD, her daughter quietly asked her about the anger issues. After discussing it, the nurse practitioner told the patient that she was allowed to get angry sometimes, especially in middle school.

5 WORDS
RILEY ERIKSEN (PRE-CLINICAL JULY 2023)

In the psychiatric unit, I watched the medical student on rotation perform a memory test on a patient. The patient easily drew a clock and identified the animals drawn, however when it came time to repeat the 5 words the student listed, she could only remember 3. "I hate to say I can't," she said.

LIKE KIDS
RILEY ERIKSEN (PRE-CLINICAL JULY 2023)

"They're like kids," the doctor said after calling a patient who didn't answer. "They don't do their labs, they don't answer the phone, they don't take their medications." Later, while writing detailed directions to send home with another patient, he smiled and said, "He probably won't read them but at least we're trying our best."

FATIGUE
RILEY ERIKSEN (PRE-CLINICAL JULY 2023)

A patient came into the office complaining of fatigue. He was anemic, taking metformin, and had atrial fibrillation. When he asked the doctor why he was so tired, he explained that it may not be just one thing. The doctor ordered an iron study, vitamin B12 panel, and talked about the possibility of cardiac ablation.

NOT THE PROBLEM
RILEY ERIKSEN (PRE-CLINICAL JULY 2023)

During rounds, we checked on a patient with dementia. As we told her and her husband she could go home, they discussed scheduling a follow-up appointment. When we said they could schedule it for the afternoon in case mornings are difficult, the patient laughed, pointed at her husband, and said she wouldn't be the problem.

SCUBA DIVING
MEGHAN CAWOOD (PRE-CLINICAL JULY 2023)

Chief complaint: "something came up while scuba diving". I followed the doctor into the room and saw a man sitting there who looked confused. He had developed two cysts on his perineum one day before his scuba trip. Amazingly soaking in the sea for hours at a time actually helped the inflammation resolve.

C+
MEGHAN CAWOOD (PRE-CLINICAL JULY 2023)

"You get a C+ for holding still," the doctor says. I'm getting a knee injection to relieve some pain I've had now for a while. After hip replacements and shoulder surgery, my body has been through the ringer. Yet, it's hard to hold still when there is a needle being shoved into my knee.

WHAT IS IT CALLED?
MEGHAN CAWOOD (PRE-CLINICAL JULY 2023)

I sit and stare into the distance. I don't know why I am here. People with badges and clipboards are always walking around. An older lady sits at a table next to me playing a game with red and black disks on a square board. Seems familiar, but I cannot remember what it is called.

SHOUT FOR JOY
MEGHAN CAWOOD (PRE-CLINICAL JULY 2023)

I wait nervously as the scans are pulled up. Doc says my tumor has grown 2 cm more, but I'm ecstatic because it hasn't metastasized! My daughter and I shout for joy! This is the best news, I exclaim. I can't do surgery because of my lungs, but chemo and radiation I can do… and I will!

AWAKE
MEGHAN CAWOOD (PRE-CLINICAL JULY 2023)

I ask for something for my anxiety. I'm laying on an operating table awake, waiting for the doctor to come in. I have had this cardiac loop recorder for 7 years now, it was only supposed to be there for one year, and today they are removing it. But I'm awake during the procedure and very scared.

NOT MY PROBLEM
EMILY AMYX (PRE-CLINICAL JULY 2023)

Before leaving the room, the patient asked me my age. "23" I stated. She laughed and said, "I thought you were 16, you look so young." I replied, "I know, it's a problem". She ended the encounter with a joyful "Well I wish I had that problem, so you can just shut the hell up".

WHAT'S THE REAL STORY?
EMILY AMYX (PRE-CLINICAL JULY 2023)

"Maybe I'm not asking the right questions" I say as we leave the room of a patient who gave a different story to the APRN than me. "Don't beat yourself up. I've had patients tell my MA's they have no concerns while having a heart attack. They give information to who they want" she replied.

TIME MATTERS
EMILY AMYX (PRE-CLINICAL JULY 2023)

"Sir, the only reason you are alive is because of that machine in your chest, you cannot wait years to come see me next. This is very important" the doctor explained. Before the encounter he told me that he has not seen this man since he placed the ICD. That was 3 years ago.

WHO AM I?
EMILY AMYX (PRE-CLINICAL JULY 2023)

"Let me know if he gives you trouble" the doctor explained. "He is usually okay but sometimes he's mean. His wife is very ill and it's really frustrating for him." I walk in the room cautiously and before I shut the door behind me, the patient belts out "Now who the hell are you?"

CHAPTER 10

Through a Rural Lens

A NORTHERN GIRL WITH A COUNTRY CALLING MARIA SHIELDS (PRE-MATRIC JULY 2020)

Mrs. B spent her first moments of life travelling through the bustling streets of Chicago. Born prematurely at 7 1/2 months with a heart murmur, it wasn't long before hospital staff ordered her transfer to another hospital for more specialized care. Not long after her birth, she laid inside of an incubator - in the backseat of a taxi cab. Under a nurse's careful supervision, she laid in the taxi whirring through the streets toward the place that would afford her a chance at life.

Mrs. B continued travelling throughout her life. She grew up in the northwest suburbs of Chicago with her parents with whom she is very close. While her parents have lived in Chicago for over 40 years, Mrs. B made the decision to move to Kentucky in 2002. She found herself in Western Kentucky in a small town where she claims everybody cares for one another. She claims that's what it's like in small communities - neighbors supporting neighbors in times of need. She says this is even more important now with the threat of COVID-19 among other social issues taking place in our communities and nation at large. She occasionally returns to her northern home where many ask her where she went. They say she has developed a southern drawl, although Mrs. B doesn't think so. Although she moved temporarily to the larger city of Louisville, she claimed that she missed country life in "The Berg", as she calls it. She thinks this urge for small town life is just in her "soul, system, and blood".

She works at the local Kroger where she has a physically demanding job that influenced her visit to the clinic today. She has bilateral knee pain and swelling that she believes is part of the "wear and tear" that her job has created over the years. She recalls working since she was 19 years old, aside from the two years during which she gave birth to her three children. She has worked every day since the onset of the novel coronavirus pandemic before she took a 12-day vacation to northwestern Indiana with her daughter's aunt, uncle, and their children. They travelled to the beach where she claimed the water was too cold to go in, but she still had a great time with her family. She claims that 90% of the cars in the parking lots had Illinois license plates where the quarantine hadn't yet been lifted. She didn't realize how much she needed the vacation. She says she quickly realized how burnt out she was. Mrs. B is a believer of taking care of herself. She insists that she must be healthy herself in order to properly care for her children.

Family is very important to Mrs. B. She is a single mother to three children that she loves dearly. She says sometimes things are hard financially as she struggles to receive child support from her daughter's father. She joyfully reflected on her decision not to marry him. Through this hardship, she is inseparable from her youngest daughter who she says is her "sidekick and shadow". She wants her daughter to go to college so that she can have a good life; one even better than this life that her parents gave her. Outside of her busy work schedule, she takes classes at a local community college with the goal to obtain an Associate Degree in Applied Sciences. She claimed she will be just like the receptionist at this clinic in the work she will do.

Mrs. B recognizes the value of every person and believes that every person's life matters. She believes it is difficult for some people to see the big picture of life and believes that everyone should try to be more open-minded. She even explains this to others in her own community where she advocates this idea. Overall, Mrs. B believes she has had a good life. She is appreciative of the care she receives from her family physician and speaks highly of her personality and ability to relate to her patients. According to Mrs. B, "She is not only my doctor, but she is also my friend." Because of this, Mrs. B says she is always honest with her physician and trusts her recommendations. Outside of her trusted family physician, Mrs. B speaks highly of physicians like her who are personable and approachable.

A RETIRED GRANDMOTHER AND TALENTED CERAMIST
MARIA SHIELDS (PRE-MATRIC JULY 2020)

Life was simpler when Mrs. W was a young girl. Her family was the first on their block to get a TV. She'll never forget the rambunctious kids and neighbors racing by to catch a peak at the glowing box of wonder. When not glued to the TV, she spoke of sweltering afternoons when she would play outside in the dirt with her siblings - hands void of electronics, trading cell phones for soil. On the weekends, she would attend "sock hops" at the youth center across the street from her beloved high school. As a child, she remembers that she much preferred to read about history and the nation's past rather than fumble with mathematics.

After Mrs. W had three children of her own, she sewed most of their clothing throughout their early childhood. She only made pants for her son though, since she could hardly ever get him to wear a shirt. After Mrs. W retired, she took up ceramics as a hobby that allowed her to create masterpieces for those she loved. For the past 12 years, she has repeated the careful process of sculpting, firing, painting, and glazing. As if in awe of her prowess, staring back at her stood sets of deer, a litter of puppies, and an owl, among her other creations. She claims the eyes were always the hardest step of the sculpting process, requiring great concentration and precision.

Before she retired, Mrs. W worked at the local hospital for 20 years. She reminisces on her past 43 years working for the public with great joy and appreciation. Mrs. W was born in Evansville but spent most of her childhood and life in Western Kentucky - and has no intentions of leaving. Not only do her 19 grandchildren and 6 great grandchildren need her here, she says, "It's just home." Mrs. W values the small-town atmosphere and the people of Western Kentucky. She spent the past four years in Pennsylvania which she claims has been a far stretch from her country home.

Mrs. W grew up in a time when tuberculosis was a common cause of death. As a young girl, her father was admitted to Chicago's tuberculosis hospital. Although her father passed when she was only 10 years old, she vividly remembers the two years he remained hospitalized. Years later, her step father passed away from a stroke when she was 16 years old. As Mrs. W grew older, she lost her sister, brother, and mother. Her first husband and father of her children passed 23 years ago after battling a plethora of health issues. She warned to "never judge a book by its cover" and to be kind to everyone. She recalls several occasions when coworkers would question why her children's father would spend most of his time at home. They wondered and accused. Why didn't he work or get out of the house? He was the picture of health, but little did they know that behind closed doors he was suffering from various health issues. Mrs. W says that everyone has a story - and you never know what their story entails.

Mrs. W's family has a large mistrust of physicians after the death of a loved one under the care of a trusted cardiologist who they claim contributed to his passing. Despite this and the great loss she has experienced, she sits in the office today obtaining a Medicare wellness visit with the company of her daughter. Mrs. W says her children are concerned about her health - especially after the discovery of a problem in her heart. Mrs. W understands this, but she believes it is best not to dwell on this. She claims that it "could always be worse" and that she is thankful for her remaining health. Her life philosophy is simple - smile, be kind, and give respect to everyone you encounter.

COVID IS JUST ONE MORE OBSTACLE –
EMILY BOLINGER (CRS JULY 2020)

Last week, I wrote about how the rural community did not suffer much consequence with the requirement of masks. This week it still holds true. The dated familiarity of patients with their doctor makes it easy to forget that masks are even a factor, but one factor has affected patients: travel. Patients in rural communities often have to travel to see a specialist and with them being sick, it creates great risk of exposure. For some, the risk of exposure is greater than the treatment provided. Of course, this makes sense, but the situation might be different if the array of specialties were as available to rural communities as they are in cities. Although it is improving, patients are often referred out of town to get the help they need. But how can they when covid-19 is on the rise? It is a challenge and a disadvantage. One patient, who previously was diagnosed with ovarian cancer but recovered, has been going to her oncologist in Texas every few months. She had to push back her appointment because the risk of getting exposed to the virus was too great. She seemed a little distressed by this but was comforted by the fact that her blood work results looked normal.

Being from a rural community myself, I understand the lack of specialty care. The woman with ovarian cancer has to travel through many states. With the pandemic on the rise, the accessibility to specialties is needed now more than ever. The point of saying all this is to bring attention to the overbearing weight of a global pandemic and its effect on rural communities who are at a major disadvantage. One issue has been around for centuries, the other, less than a year. The difference is one will be fought by a vaccine, and the other, is at a much slower progression. I truly hope the pandemic resolves quickly, but much more than that I hope that it teaches us that the need is urgent. I hope everyone gets the care they need, and I hope that a trip to Texas will soon become a trip into town.

LIVING THE SIMPLE LIFE–EMILY BOLINGER (CRS JULY 2020)

When I met this woman, I could tell by her cowgirl boots that she is a local. When I heard her accent to match, I knew we had a gal that grew up here. She told me she was born and raised in Greenville, and she was on the Greenville High School basketball team. That is when she was diagnosed with epilepsy. I could tell by the look in her eyes that this has been a struggle her whole life. She is thirty-four years old. She has been married for thirteen years, and she has three kids. She used to work at the minute mart in her younger years, but now she "works with all boys, all day". She does plumbing, electric, and other kinds of vocational work. She boasted that she is "not afraid to get her hands dirty". She said she is a country girl as she called attention to her cowgirl boots. She laughed, but I could hear the pride in her voice. She is a small-town girl. She the youngest…the "brat" as she called herself. I related to this because I also am the youngest, and my older sister never lets me forget it. Growing up in a small town myself, I have known many girls like her. I am even like her in some ways. The word I use to describe people like this is content. They are satisfied with their life just as it is. The do not get caught up on things that city folk want. The slow and family-oriented life is what this woman was born to live.

The last question I asked her was "What advice do you have for me as a future doctor?" She sat back and thought about it. "Never give up. And do not forget your bedside manner!" We laughed together, and parted ways. This was such simple advice. I thought for sure she would have a laundry list for me. But then I thought, 'This exactly sums this woman up…simple'. It also sums up how many people live in rural communities. This is not to put down these people. I actually admire this characteristic. If there is one thing I learned from this woman, it is that there is absolutely nothing wrong with being from/living in a small town. There is actually something to say for who live simple and content. We could all learn this lesson

NO ONE'S RIGHT AND NO ONE'S WRONG
JORDAN HARBIN (CRS JULY 2021)

I know your family; y'all will be fine.

Multi-system organ failure has put him on dialysis.

I know where I got the covid, my boy.

He smiled as he pondered his chances of getting a transplant.

He said his son wasn't allowed to come in the house anymore,

Politics. No right or wrong. Serenity prayer.

MASKS DON'T MATTER
EMILY BOLINGER (CRS JULY 2020)

Recently, I had the opportunity to shadow a rural physician. With the COVID-19 pandemic at hand, I was fortunate to get to experience first-hand the effects of such an event. Therefore, in an office where only half of every face is visible, you expect a substantial social affect. I arrived at the shadowing site, had my temperature taken, and was directed to my assigned wing of the outpatient facility. As I met everyone in the internal medicine unit, I assured them I was smiling under the mask. They gave a laugh at that. Soon after my tour, I met my preceptor, and we started seeing patients. All patients were under the same regimen. They had their temperature taken and were properly masked. From room to room, I witnessed the interactions between patient and doctor. I realized nothing has changed. Patients are still able to see their doctors and get their treatments. Likewise, patients have maintained their relationship with their doctor. One benefit to rural medicine is having ties to your patient. You usually have a relationship with them. This was not affected by required masks. Doctors still connected as normal with their patients. I contribute this to the established familiarity of the patient to the doctor pre-pandemic.

One encounter, specifically, showed me the power of rural medicine despite the boundaries at hand. My preceptor walked into a room to an elderly woman to whom she was delivering bad news. They greeted one another, as did I, and the doc sat in her chair and positioned herself so that she was face to face with her patient. I witnessed the personal conversation they had while this patient realized that mortality was at hand. It was emotional. It was empathetic. It was unaffected by the masks between them. Other patients had more lighthearted experiences with their doctor, and the more I witnessed, the more I realized that rural culture is stronger than a face mask. The doctor I was shadowing has an established relationship with each of her patients, so she did not need to see their whole face to connect with them. I must admit I was surprised by my findings. I expected to write an article saying, "Masks are depersonalizing the patient to doctor relationship". I guess us rural folk are just too darn stubborn to let that happen. Or maybe it is because that the connectedness of a rural community cannot be hindered as easily as places that are already disconnected. I cannot speak to how the pandemic guidelines have affected other areas or even other practices. I know for a while even the doctor I was shadowing felt a distance from her patients through the implementation of telehealth. All I can attest to is what I saw that day which was a doctor who was connecting to patients that trusted her.

CHAPTER 11

The Depth of Human Misery

THOSE KIDS ARE ROTTEN
WILLIAM J. CRUMP, MD

One of my current missions is to try to assist medical students and residents as they develop their professional identity. My goal is to make them a little less cynical. My favorite definition of a cynic is someone who cannot imagine anyone else being motivated by anything but self- interest.

I also wish to inoculate them against severe burnout. The definition of burnout that I like the best is that it is a dislocation between what you thought you would be doing and what you actually end up doing. Another favorite description is that burnout is "erosion of the soul" that leads to ill health, depression, dissociation from important relationships and a downward spiral of worsening cynicism.

One of the exercises I do with my learners is to have them recall a situation where they clearly had one opinion and understanding of a patient that was dramatically different once the "rest of the story" was known. I have them actually draw a comic with word balloons over the sketched characters, describing their understanding of the before and after versions of the patient stories.

As I did this comic drawing exercise myself, I recalled three women who I had seen recently in my role as medical support of our inpatient behavioral health unit, all admitted to the hospital for suicidal ideation, none on the unit at the same time. All three were angry with the world and each had new superficial linear lacerations on their arms that spoke to the need to feel something.

When taking their social and family history, each really focused on the disrespect shown them by their biological children, all teenagers. When I also asked as I always do about contraception, each said emphatically "Don't need any." So as always, I responded "So you're not having sexual intercourse?" Each responded negatively with some version of "Never again." All three of the women reported having current female partners.

I am often within earshot as the unit group sessions begin, and I overheard each of these women very angrily telling others about their kids. One said that she couldn't care less about her kids, and another said she didn't give a s - - - what happened to her kids. Each used some version of calling them "rotten," and each didn't care if she never saw them again.

So I made some assumptions about these women. The new partners were part of the household now, and I could imagine that unruly teenagers might not be entirely sensitive to their current situation and this behavior might actually make them feel more disconnected and hopeless.

None of the three stayed in the unit long enough for me to get to know them better. It was only in talking with the staff later that I discovered "the rest of the story." The story each patient told, confirmed by other family members, was that these children were the result of repeated rapes. One was by a step-father, one by an uncle, and one, especially troubling, was by her biological father.

These, and so many other stories from everyday practice, continually cause me to reflect and reconsider many assumptions. Humans can do bad things to each other, and my job is still to try to dispense hope every chance I get. Maybe by listening empathetically, our staff helped these women in some small way. Maybe each will share more in time with their outpatient therapist now that each has revealed it to the behavioral health staff. Some wounds don't begin to heal until the scab is off, I guess. And maybe the next time a physician sets aside cynicism and approaches them with genuine empathy, they will receive some solace. At least, that's my hope.

A FLAW IN HER PLAN
CIERRA WOODCOCK (PRE-MATRIC JUNE 2021)

Mrs. T was a 63-year old woman hospitalized for an attempted suicide via overdose. Prior to attempting suicide, Mrs. T spent $1000 purchasing jewels for a game called "Fishdom" on her iPhone. She suffered from a multitude of mental health issues including anxiety, depression, post-traumatic stress disorder, and an impulse control disorder. She was begging to go home, but earlier that morning she had gotten in a fight with another patient over sharing a purple marker and had gotten unreasonably angry when the psychiatrist told her she did not need some of the medicines she had been taking. Her mood changes were so sporadic, that by the time I got to interview her, she was happy and complimenting my dress.

Mrs. T immediately began to cry when asked to tell her story, beginning with early childhood. She began by stating that of all her siblings, her father chose to only beat her. He beat her for any small mistake she made, for doing things with her brothers, but mostly for no particular reason at all. She described the horrendous verbal and physical abuse she experienced from her father, including how he called her vulgar names and hit her in the face with his belt buckle until her face was black and blue. However, the worst part of her story was not the beatings, it was the sexual abuse. She claimed that when she was only 15, her father snuck into her room late one night and raped her. He thought she would stay asleep, but she woke up to discover him touching her inappropriately. As he raped her, she stayed silent. She was more afraid of what he would do to her if anyone found out. Later on, her father and his friends gang-raped her. They made her perform oral sex on them and laughed as she cried out in pain. They spit on her and told her "this is what women are supposed to do." This happened when she was only 16. She remained silent about the incident for years in fear that her father would do much worse than the heinous actions he had previously committed.

To escape her father, she married her first husband after only knowing him for six weeks. She claimed that her leaving triggered her mother's nervous breakdown and she did not get out of bed for a month. Her mother was devastated that she married so young because she wanted her to go to college to become a nurse and assumed she wouldn't go to school now that she was married. However, Mrs. T did become a nurse and eventually worked three jobs to support her daughter and her grandchildren until 2004. It was at this point she found out that her granddaughter had also been sexually assaulted by her father. Here, she shared her story with her granddaughter to show her that she was not alone and she was going to be there to help her in any way she could. Eventually, her daughter cut ties with her and would no longer allow her to see her granddaughter. Her mother, who was also her best friend, passed away shortly after. This triggered the oncoming of severe depression and previous traumatic events getting the best of Mrs. T's mental health. This was when she discussed the plotting of her own death.

Lastly, Mrs. T told me exactly how she planned to end her own life and ultimately how she ended up in the psychiatric unit. She began by stating that she was going to take a shower to get herself as clean as possible. She was then going to put on a new outfit, fill the tub with hot water, and then slit her wrists with razor blades. She even said that she took all of her Tylenol III pills so they would thin her blood so she would bleed to death quickly. She claimed that her only flaw was calling her daughter right before she carried out her plan and that is how she ended up in the hospital. Honestly, I believe what she considered to be a "flaw" in her plan was actually a cry for help.

GRIEF
SHAINA MAGNESS (CRS JULY 2021)

She takes high-dose Xanax three times a day just to get by.

She was anxious before, but it was never this bad.

When her daughter suddenly died, she lost a vital part of herself.

She can't sleep, she can't work, and she can't be herself anymore.

She is getting better with the medication, but she needs more than Dr. W can provide.

She is 36th in line for psychiatry.

SHE SAVED HIM
LAUREN TROUT (CRS JULY 2022)

His daughter just turned a week old. Being a new parent may have been his stressor. He writes in a journal to find his peace. A story about his daughter and how she saved him was shared with the group- she is his moon. His purpose was found in her. But yet, he is here

FOR BETTER OR FOR WORSE
MEGHAN CAWOOD (PRE-MATRIC JUNE 2020)

I was born and raised in Madisonville, KY. My childhood was actually terrible, as I vividly remember waking up when I was a kid and hating my life. Everything was dark and scary. I have one sister who is younger than me and we never got along. Life seemed pretty hopeless and then to top it off one terrible morning my mom left and we were alone. Our father was already out of the picture, and it was just my sister at age 10 and I at age 12. The best thing that could have happened and did in fact happen was my aunt taking us in. She was really fun, kind, and supportive and she would take us on trips to Florida in the summertime.

When I turned 16 years old, I began working in the fast-food business and have done that ever since. While I finished high school I never went onto college as my fast-food job was enough for me. I was married for 19 years before divorcing the man and I just got married again this year to a new fella. However, my new husband is never there for me, and even now while I sit in the hospital trying to reach him, he continues to ignore me and refuses to pick up the phone. They say, "For better or for worse" and he is definitely pushing my relationship into more of 'the worse' side of the scale. As for children, I have a 20-year-old son, who is a good guy, and he loves to drive cars and go fast. He even takes me for rides in my Corvette. However, my son knows he can't have friends over to the house all the time, and yet my silly husband is allowing it, so there are a bunch of teenagers in my home.

Apart from all that stuff, I do have a dog who is a mix between a Pit-bull, German shepherd, and Labrador retriever, and who I love very much. When I have free time I like to clean up his 'poo', but on a more serious note, I like to take him to the dog park. But other than my dog, I don't have any other hobbies or things I like to do. My plan for when I get out of the hospital is to get back to work and get stuff done. As for a trait that is unique to me that I think everybody should know is that I am funny and I like to laugh.

THE STRONG ONE
HANNAH TURNER (PRE-MATRIC JUNE 2023)

Holding strong for one's family is a monumental task. Ms. F shouldered the weight of this early in life and carried it for years. Eventually, it became her identity. When I met her, she was lying on her bed in the inpatient psychiatric ward. Her tangled dark hair stuck out in every direction, and her shoulders slumped forward as she rolled to a sitting position. Her sadness was palpable before she even spoke. She honored my intrusion with some of her story.

As a little girl, she had been powerless to stop her father from physically abusing her mom. When she grew "big enough to fight back," she protected her mom. This early trauma followed her into adulthood. Her primary purposes in life became protecting and caring for others.

Her mom's death in 2020 brought Ms. F's world to a screeching halt. Along with her mother, she had lost her purpose. "I just don't have a purpose anymore, nobody needs me" she lamented throughout the interview. As she lifted her flat eyes to meet mine, they emanated hopelessness. Her mom was gone, her siblings were independent, and her boyfriend was self-sufficient. She no longer felt needed. The day before we spoke, she had attempted suicide by a gabapentin overdose. Her boyfriend had rushed her to the hospital. The only activity offering her solace was fishing, a pastime begun in childhood. My heart ached for Ms. F as I heard her story.

As we spoke, I wondered what it be like to feel what she was feeling? I searched for the right words to comfort her, to convince her of her value, to instill hope. The right words wouldn't come. I knew they wouldn't fix it, but wished they would. I could only offer Ms. F a listening ear. When I think of Ms. F, I am reminded that even the strongest people need help sometimes.

ONE DAY AT A TIME
ALEC TAYLOR (PRE-MATRIC JUNE 2023)

Ms. W's perfect day consists of fishing with her boyfriend and going home to watch a NASCAR race on television afterward. On occasion, she travels to Bristol to watch the cars zoom around the track. Even though she admits it probably isn't healthy for her hearing, she loves hearing the roaring engines. Although she loves the simple things in life, life circumstances have made it difficult to enthrall herself in these things.

She was born to a 26-year-old African American mother and a 50-year-old Caucasian father. Her father previously fathered six, all Caucasian, children with another woman. For the entirety of her life, her siblings ignored and ostracized her from family events. Ms. W had to deal with her mother passing away young and the pressure of caring for her father in his elderly years.

Three years ago, her father passed away in his early eighties. Not surprisingly, her siblings did not support her during the mourning of her father. Only having short, dry conversations with them during the funeral, she doesn't have any family left on her paternal side. Thankfully, she still had her maternal grandmother.

However, her grandmother also grew elderly and passed away three months ago. With no family left, Ms. W only has her boyfriend. Although her boyfriend struggled with drug addiction in the past, he sobered up and became the focal point of her support system. Ms. W admits that her boyfriend has been instrumental in this healing process, but she cannot bear the weight of her life circumstances.

Now on the psychiatry unit, Ms. W has been diagnosed with major depressive disorder. Most days she does not have an appetite, and she tosses and turns when attempting to sleep at night. She makes up for her restless nights during the day when she isn't exploding with tearful emotions. The healing process takes time, but Ms. W eagerly wants to return to her normal life. One day at a time, she will do anything necessary to recover from the effects of her unfortunate life events. She said she might even buy a new fishing pole when she gets out.

In retrospect, my experience with Ms. W enlightened me more than any textbook. As someone lucky enough to come from a stable household, I had never engaged in a long conversation with someone about their family trauma. When I envisioned individuals checking into a psychiatric unit, I concentrated on their potential disorders, not their stories. Life dealt many of these individuals an unfortunate hand. Some of these patients' life circumstances never gave them a chance to develop their minds. Discerning a patient's story may be imperative in all medical specialties, yet the story seemed crucially fundamental on this unit due to the severity of the trauma. I will try to hone the skill of obtaining the story throughout my career, and I will recall my interview with Ms. W to remind myself of the utmost importance of the patient narrative, no matter the heaviness of the tale.

DOUBLE WIDOW
IAN LEATHERMAN (CRS JULY 2023)

The conversation began with an introduction of myself to the patient from the third year medical student. The medical school student stated that I was working on a project for a summer program and then turned it over to me. I began by introducing myself a bit more to the patient and then telling her that the premise of my project was to discover aspects of patient life which are unknown to their doctors. She immediately began telling me about how she ended up in the situation she was currently in. From what I gathered, she had been prescribed medicines that were contraindicatory to each other, causing her to have schizophrenic-like symptoms, such as hallucinations. She mentioned that the first person to notice she was acting differently was her daughter with whom she had a very close relationship. She stated that she thought she was acting completely normal, and that she was so thankful that her daughter cared enough about her to seek help. This prompted me to ask about if she had any other kids, which brought our interview into territory that I was definitely not expecting.

She said that her daughter was from her first husband, and that she had two sons from her second husband. She followed this up by telling me she was a double widow. I responded by asking if she would feel comfortable telling me about how it all happened. She said she didn't mind and started telling me about her first husband. He was an abusive alcoholic, who passed away due to his alcoholism. As she began telling me about her second husband I could see her eyes begin to fill up with tears. Her second husband was a Gulf War Veteran. She said that shortly after they got married he was diagnosed with brain cancer. They were married for 8 years before he eventually passed. She explained that in the Gulf War he was exposed to a bunch of chemicals which is what caused his cancer. She talked about how they first met: He knocked on her door and told her, not asked her, to come over and try his gumbo (he was from Louisiana). By the end of her explaining the ins and outs of her marriages, her glasses were on the table, and she had tears coming down both cheeks. I was floored, and frankly, I didn't really know the right thing to say. I responded with the first thing that came to mind, "Thank you for telling me your story, you are obviously a very strong woman." She smiled, wiped her eyes, and thanked me.

I asked her if she had ever told her doctors what she had just told me. Because she was a patient in the psychiatry unit, I figured she had definitely brought these things up previously to her doctors but she said she couldn't remember if she had or not. "Do you think that this is something they should know?" I responded. "Well. they have never asked me about any of this," she returned.

I felt that we had talked about her marriage enough and I wanted to switch the conversation to a more positive topic. I remarked that she had been through a lot in her life, and questioned where she sees her life going as she moves forward. She explained that she wants to focus on being healthy and being with her family. She wants to move closer to her daughter so she can see her and her grandchildren more. She explained that she also wanted to move because her landlord had found out about the pension she received from her second husband's death and told her that he was going to increase her rent. She explained this as being a blessing in disguise because she had wanted to move closer to her daughter for a while anyways. She said that she also wants to focus on her grandchildren being healthy. She explained that she had dealt with drug addiction early in her life, and the last thing she wanted was for her grandchildren to go through that too. The last statement she made regarding her future was that she wants her communication with her doctors and the other people helping her take care of her health to be more clear. Obviously, ending up in the hospital because of medications she had been taking was something she wanted to avoid in the future.

I concluded the conversation by stating, "I am an aspiring doctor, and I want to finish off this conversation by asking you if you have any advice for me." She responded by telling me how important it is to listen and take my time. Furthermore, she emphasized how important it is to build and maintain the relationships I have with patients.

Overall, this patient interview was both eye opening and inspiring. To hear about such hardship and have the person who experienced all of it right in front of me was a first. It was an experience that I will never forget. Her story was filled with many valleys. She had fought through drug addiction, abuse, and the death of not one, but two spouses. Yet, she was still present and taking time out of her day to help a student with his project. As she was breaking down and laying out such personal information about her life, I had to hold back tears of my own. I knew that I was not supposed to cry in front of a patient. But, I didn't want to hide my compassion from her either—that I was feeling what she was feeling. Thinking back on the interaction now, I wonder why she felt so comfortable being vulnerable with me as someone who has no expertise in the field of psychiatry, someone who hasn't even earned a college degree. Maybe it isn't simply a doctor's credentials that make a good doctor, maybe it is simply the ability to ask good questions and be a good listener.

VERY LUCKY SURVIVOR
ISAAC KREBS (CRS JULY 2023)

Mr. X is a 20-year-old on the hospital Psychiatry unit. A very talkative and laidback guy, he shared with me so many things. He has a dog, a 6-year-old little sister back in Illinois, where he grew up, and a grandmother in Kentucky. He lived with his mother for a while and she was mostly unemployed with odd jobs along the way. His childhood became tragic early as his mother beat him, smoked weed around him, and generally treated him badly. She left him early in life. As a kid in school, he loved learning about history. He ended up with a GED after being suspended from multiple schools. His troubles with drugs started early, as he started smoking weed at age 10. He eventually moved to harder drugs, getting to the point with fentanyl that morphine drips did nothing to him. As abuse mounted, he ran away, only accepted by drug houses so that even he realized," [Its] all about the environment you're in". He cut his arms frequently, thinking about death more and more as he approached 20. He also got a girlfriend somewhere along this journey, who shared his pills. He also was in jail at some point, where he tried to hang himself. There ended up being a warrant out for them and the relationship ended when they overdosed. They haven't seen each other since. He then went to a rehab program where he reported that he was sexually assaulted. He was then admitted to this hospital, where he has been for 16 days.

When I asked about his hobbies, he focused on shooting basketball and hiking as his favorites, loving Land Between the Lakes, Shawnee Forest in Illinois, and Garden of the Gods. His favorite food is Chinese. I asked him what would need to happen for him to get better, and he responded that he would need to think about death far less often. He thinks of himself as a very lucky survivor, which is a thing of pride for him.

I was blown away by his story because I had never talked to anyone who had actually seen a lot of the worst America holds. It was enlightening to talk with him and see his humanity through his pain, and I appreciated the opportunity to be with him as he recounted his life.

HOW CAN I MAKE FRIENDS
MEGHAN CAWOOD (PRE-CLINICAL JULY 2023)

I was born in Albuquerque in 1960. I grew up in a terrible household in which my three brothers and I were beaten by belts and sticks. My mother was not only physically abusive, but also verbally, constantly telling me that I should be dead and that I am totally useless. My father, however, was my hero. He used to work so hard and was always there when I needed him. He let me ride his horses and play with his pets. When I was a teenager we moved to Illinois which is the one place where I really began to make great friends. We would have sleepovers with movies and popcorn all the time. My best friends and I really enjoyed the Nicholas Sparks movies. I also really enjoyed swimming and playing tennis with them too.

I got married when I was young, moved to Western Kentucky, and had two beautiful children, one boy and one girl. I used to do everything with them like taking them for ice cream or putt-putt. To make money for my family I became a CNA at a nursing home which was very enjoyable because I was able to take my daughter to work with me. Life was going really well until fights with my husband started. My marriage ended when my husband told me he wanted me to die and pushed me down the stairs. I broke my back and knee cap and am now on disability because of it. To make matters worse, a few years back my older brother committed suicide, and a year ago my son died of a heart condition. This just broke me. Love is so special and when you lose the ones you love and the ones that love you, it's the worst feeling in the world. I became very depressed and thought about killing myself this past Christmas. A few weeks ago my daughter needed $1000 and I gave it to her, but it left me short on my rent and I was kicked out of my home. I have spent the last few days at the shelter, but I have no friends and feel completely alone. Can you tell me how I can make some friends?

This story was very difficult to hear as you could tell that it really hurt the patient to relive some of her past. She would get very tearful talking about her relationship with her mother and the death of her son. Aside from the stories she told she showed true kindness which made me sad as she kept emphasizing her loneliness. I felt as though I wanted to keep talking to her and asking her questions to show that someone cared and was willing to spend the time listening.

A SOUTHERN WOMAN WITH A SPUNKY SOUL
MARIA SHIELDS (M4, AUGUST 2023)

Our rural psychiatry unit received a voluntary admission of a female patient in her 30s for suicidal ideation. Upon her arrival, I had the pleasure of meeting Harley (not her real name) - a young woman from the south, who found herself in an abusive relationship involving drug use. She spoke highly of her brother, who she says saved her from this relationship and enabled her to move to the area to live with him. Most recently, he paid a deposit to a local recovery center to get treatment for her methamphetamine use disorder and mental illness. After arrival at the center, Harley endorsed suicidal ideation – she identified no plan but wondered what the world would "be like without her" and questioned, "Why am I here?"

As more of the story unfolded, she revealed "problems with the staff" and felt that she didn't fit in. She endorsed many obstacles preventing her from getting a job, stable housing, or an income to cover mental health medications. I attempted to put myself in her shoes and was discouraged by how impossible and far away these goals felt. Ultimately, she remained intensely focused on convincing her brother that she didn't need rehab. We talked with Harley about internalizing control of her situation and identifying her own values and aligning her actions with those. She seemingly had a breakthrough and insisted that upon discharge that day, she would return to the recovery center.

The following Monday, I saw an unhappy Harley being rolled into the unit. Numerous questions raced through my mind – "Did something happen at the recovery center?", "Did she want to be back here?" She expressed that upon return to the recovery center, she "starved". They would not provide money for her medications, and she had to eat out of a community box which made her feel "less than". She expressed that if she went back to the recovery center, she would try to commit suicide because of the "way they are" and that "it's their fault". On the other hand, Harley confided that she felt particularly connected to some of the staff members of our unit because she believed they were "spunky" like her. During her first admission, her brother denied her request to come home, and suddenly he became the persecutor for doing so. I started to put together the pieces and began to witness Harley's black-and-white thinking – all or nothing. Everyone was either all good or all bad – there was no "in-between". An individual's designation into either category was based on their level of support of her situation at the moment and if she could relate to them.

At first, it was difficult not to see Harley as a helpless victim in need of saving. I reflected on the rest of her story – a childhood in the foster care system and countless experiences of physical, verbal, sexual, and emotional abuse. Harley was undoubtedly a victim of indescribable suffering and had subsequently developed maladaptive ways of navigating the world, demonstrated through her cluster B personality traits and borderline personality disorder. I grappled with the idea that her BPD, emotional dysregulation, and ineffective coping were an outward representation of the inner work that young Harley did to cope with the chaotic world and trauma around her.

As a medical student, I found myself eager to play a role in Harley's care. On her first day in the unit, she approached the nurse's station and asked me for help with calling her brother. My preceptor quickly encouraged me to be cautious about requests like these as we discussed the dynamics of "Karpman's triangle" involving a persecutor, victim, and rescuer. How easy it can be for us, especially those who find purpose and meaning in helping others, to fall into Karpman's drama triangle. Not recognizing my unleashed empathy, I found myself, unknowingly, about to step into the role of "rescuer" in the triangle. Instead, I made a conscious effort to place myself within the triangle, almost as if being an "observer" of the dynamics. Surprisingly, I saw Harley take responsibility for some of her actions. Once she realized that there was no "rescuer", she began to take the initiative and make informed, educated decisions for herself. Making decisions or doing tasks for her would've only worsened the dependency and externalization of control. I came to accept that the best thing I could do for the patient at that moment was nothing - I could support her, but I couldn't do the work for her. Harley needed the support of our treatment team, but she did not need a "rescuer".

After this patient encounter, I found myself evaluating many of the personal relationships in my own life. How many times had I tried to play the role of "rescuer" in a situation, contributing to Karpman's triangle? Harley fundamentally changed the way I think about healing and serving patients and was a reminder that empathy, when harnessed, is a powerful tool that deserves a place in medicine. I learned that harnessing my empathy and letting a patient make their own autonomous decisions, even when they find themselves in a bad situation is not only useful but necessary. In my future practice, I hope that I will recognize Karpman's dynamics and guide/support my patient through their struggles without stepping into the rescuer role and potentially becoming the persecutor in the eyes of my patient. I also hope that one day Harley will see her inner strength and value – perhaps with the correct outpatient therapy and medications, she may one day even see herself as the rescuer of her own story.